A Parent's Guide to KIDNEY DISORDERS

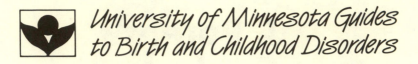

University of Minnesota Guides to Birth and Childhood Disorders

Edited by Robert J. Gorlin
Regents' Professor of Oral Pathology and Genetics
and Professor of Pediatrics, University of Minnesota

A Parent's Guide to

KIDNEY DISORDERS

Glenn H. Bock, M.D., associate professor of pediatrics at George Washington University School of Medicine and vice chairman of the Department of Pediatric Nephrology of Children's National Medical Center

Edward J. Ruley, M.D., professor of pediatrics at George Washington University School of Medicine and chairman of the Department of Pediatric Nephrology of Children's National Medical Center

and

Michael P. Moore, science writer, University of Minnesota

University of Minnesota Press
Minneapolis
London

Published by the University of Minnesota Press
2037 University Avenue Southeast, Minneapolis, MN 55455-3052
Printed in the United States of America on acid-free paper

Library of Congress Cataloging-in-Publication Data

Bock, Glenn H.
    A parent's guide to kidney disorders / Glenn H. Bock, Edward J. Ruley, and Michael P. Moore.
        p.   cm. — (University of Minnesota guides to birth and childhood disorders)
    Includes index.
    ISBN 0-8166-1745-7 (hc : acid-free paper)
    1. Pediatric nephrology–Popular works.   I. Ruley, Edward J.
II. Moore, Michael P.   III. Title.   IV. Series.
RJ176.K5B63   1993
618.92′61–dc20   92-35697
                                                                        CIP

This book is dedicated to the physicians, nurses, social workers, dietitians, and administrative staffs who are devoted to the care of children burdened with kidney diseases. The book is also dedicated to our wives and children, who patiently understand the time we must spend in providing this care.

Contents

Foreword

A Parent's Guide to Kidney Disorders is one of a series of books designed to address the needs not only of parents but also of physicians and persons concerned with the care of children with relatively common disorders. We used as a model *The Child with Down's Syndrome*, written by David W. Smith, M.D., and Ann Asper Wilson and first published in 1973 by W. B. Saunders, Philadelphia. The book is valuable because it makes the complex concepts of genetics and pediatrics understandable to parents. Such is the goal of our series.

In *A Parent's Guide to Kidney Disorders*, the authors discuss the normal functions of the kidney—that is, what the kidneys do, how these tasks are accomplished, and what happens when one or more of these functions go awry. They discuss signs and symptoms that may indicate a kidney or urinary problem, such as high blood pressure, blood and/or protein in the urine, and more subtle but significant findings such as elevated blood urea nitrogen and creatinine levels. The need for laboratory tests, radiologic studies, and, occasionally, kidney biopsy is presented in clear language. The authors have lucidly explained the more common congenital and acquired disorders of the kidney as well as discussed single-gene inheritance of several of these kidney disorders. Urinary tract infections, so common in children, are dealt with extensively. Particularly detailed description is given of chronic kidney failure, methods employed in its control, such as dialysis and transplantation, and their attendant complications. Parents will find especially helpful the discussion of psychological aspects of chronic illness in childhood and adolescence. The authors present information on the vast array of medications employed in taking care of your child, the patients' and parents' rights and responsibilities in care, and a frank discussion of costs and how financial aid may be obtained. Finally, there is a section on useful dietary guidelines.

This book was written by Glenn H. Bock, M.D., Edward J. Ruley, M.D., and Michael P. Moore. Dr. Bock has been in the field of pediatric nephrology for more than 12 years and is currently active in many aspects of professional and public education about childhood diseases of the kidney. He is vice chairman of the Department of Pediatric Nephrology of Children's National Medical Center in Washington, D.C., and is associate professor of pediatrics at George Washington University School of Medicine. Dr. Ruley is chairman of the Department of Pediatric Nephrology of Children's National Medical Center and professor of pediatrics at George Washington University School of Medicine. Drs. Bock and Ruley were chosen to write this book not only because they are excellent pediatric nephrologists but also because they have fine talents in communication. Mr. Moore has been a science writer for 10 years and is now director of communications for the Office of Research and Technology Transfer Administration at the University of Minnesota. He has also coauthored books about diabetes and epilepsy. As this book illustrates, Mr. Moore has great ability in molding highly technical material into an understandable, readable whole.

The need for this series is obvious. Parents of a child with a serious disability need answers. They need to know not only the nature of their child's disorder but also its possible causes, its prognosis, the limitations it will impose on the child, the impact it will have on the entire family, and the chances of its recurring either in the parents' future children or in the affected child's children. It is also important that parents be informed about community resources that can help them deal with the disorder. And, certainly, they need to know what they themselves can do to help.

In spite of good intentions, the health professional has not always been an effective communicator. These books are designed to open the lines of communication between the health professional and parents by increasing parents' understanding and providing them with a basic vocabulary for easier and more accurate expression of the worries, doubts, and uncertainties attendant on each disorder. It is our intention that health professionals play a vital part by supplementing each text with their own expertise. We cannot hope to answer all the questions that may be posed by parents, but we believe that each book will go a long way in answering many of the common ones.

R. J. G.

Preface

This book is written for parents of children with disorders of the kidneys and for children who are old enough to understand the information presented. We wrote it because in our experience with parents, and with many of our adolescent patients, we have found what we consider a very encouraging desire for more information about the problems affecting their lives. Having good information can help motivate parents and children to do their best to overcome a problem. As is the case with most chronic health disorders, the best results in treating kidney disorders tend to occur when patients and families are motivated to become involved in the health care process.

We find that motivation and positive involvement result when family members feel comfortable discussing concerns with their physicians and other health care providers. Most health care professionals today realize that they can be most successful when they help families work as part of a team. They do this by sharing their knowledge clearly and by involving the family in making decisions about the treatment process. Much of this information is shared through conversations during the course of diagnosis, therapy, and follow-up. We feel, however, that having a good source of written information can greatly improve the quality of communication between family members and health care professionals. We hope this book will enhance that relationship and encourage you to ask more questions and become more involved in your child's care.

Much has changed in recent years to help us make this book more useful. In fact, a book like this one, if written in the middle of the century, would have been able to provide very little information—or hope—to the parents of a child with kidney problems. For those of us who have devoted our careers to the care of children with kidney disorders, it seems incredible that the knowledge and treatments we use today were virtually nonexistent only a few decades ago.

For example, the chapters on why kidney disease occurs, how it can be diagnosed, and how it can be treated successfully would have been very short if they had been written 40 years ago. As more information has become available through research and better diagnostic tests, detection and treatment have improved. And, with the introduction of kidney dialysis, and later kidney transplantation, it became possible to help children with even the most serious kidney problems.

Just in the past decade the diagnosis and treatment of kidney diseases have changed dramatically. Doctors now have much better information and tools with which to help children with kidney disorders. Parents therefore can be realistically optimistic that their child will regain his or her good health in many settings.

The complexity of modern medicine can be overwhelming, however. There is so much information, such complex high-technology equipment, and so many tests that it is understandable that parents feel helpless and confused. Again, we hope this book will help. For example, technical terms are italicized in the text and defined in a glossary at the back of the book. And chapter 2 explains the many examinations and tests your child may have. Probably the most common complaint we hear from patients and their families is that doctors do too many tests. But if you understand why these tests are necessary, and why they sometimes must be repeated, it is a little easier to accept them as part of the path toward good health.

There is still a great need for further progress in the field of kidney disorders, especially those serious enough to require dialysis or transplantation. In chapter 11 we explain some of the recent advances and prospects for the near future. By helping to support medical research in whatever way you can, and by keeping informed about progress through your doctor or kidney organizations, you can both assist medical research and take advantage of improvements as they occur.

We hope you will use the information in this book to become an active part of your child's health care team. Or, if you are an older child reading this book, we hope it will help you see that you are not alone, and that you can be the most important person on your health care team. Either way, as an informed and motivated parent or patient, you will be one of modern medicine's greatest assets.

A Parent's Guide to KIDNEY DISORDERS

Chapter 1

The Kidneys in Health and Disease

Parents of children with kidney disorders have much to gain from a clear understanding of how the kidneys function and what can go wrong with them. Better understanding often results in greater peace of mind for parents, because rather than worrying about the unknown, they can set realistic goals and expectations for their child. This knowledge also makes parents better able to teach their child as much about the disorder as possible.

It is natural for parents to be extra protective of a child with a chronic health disorder. Although each child's health needs to be evaluated individually, in general most parents learn that their child with a kidney disorder needs very few restrictions. We have found that as parents learn more about their child's disorder, they are better able to focus on what the child can do rather than what he or she cannot do. Both the parents and the child benefit from the child's participation in play, sports, and normal activities at school to the best of his or her ability.

Education about the nature of the kidney disease may also result in better acceptance of necessary medical tests. And, it can lead to a greater commitment, on the child's part, to the treatment program.

In order to understand why and how various diseases of the kidneys occur, and why they cause certain types of problems, it is first necessary to gain some insight into the normal functions of the kidney. This chapter will introduce you to what the kidneys do, how they accomplish these tasks, and what happens when one or all of these important functions become abnormal.

The Kidneys

The human body is a complex and wonderful structure. However, its efficient operation depends on the continuous functioning of body systems that monitor and adjust the inner environment. The foremost responsibility of many body organs—including the kidneys—is to preserve this healthy environment.

The kidneys are sometimes referred to as the "chemists" of the body. They maintain water, *mineral,* and chemical balance in the body by excreting excessive amounts in the urine. When functioning normally, the kidneys have a remarkable ability to keep things in order even when we eat or drink "too much of a good thing." In order to provide energy, our bodies are always "burning" calories from the food that we eat. As a result, waste products are produced that would be harmful if not eliminated. The kidneys share a large part of the responsibility for removing these potentially harmful materials. They do this by "filtering" them from the blood and producing urine to remove them from the body.

Two of the most important factors in regulating *blood pressure* are the amount of fluid in blood vessels and the size of blood vessels (Figure 1). Both of these factors can be regulated by the kidneys. The kidneys also take active roles in stimulating the body to produce new red (oxygen-carrying) blood cells and in maintaining mineral balance and bone growth.

How the Kidneys Work

The kidneys are located on either side of the lower back, protected by muscle and ribs (Figure 2). Blood vessels called the

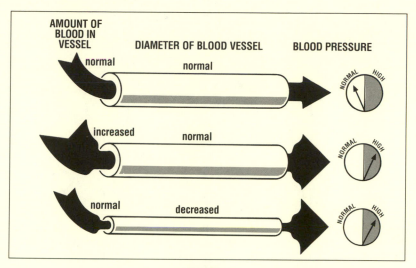

FIGURE 1

Blood pressure is controlled primarily by altering the diameter (thickness) of the blood vessels and the amount of blood flowing through them. In the *top example*, a normal blood pressure results from a balance of this size and volume. If excessive fluid is retained in the blood compartment of the body, blood pressure rises (*center drawing*). If fluid volume remains relatively normal, but the size of the blood vessel contracts (such as from hormonal signals from a diseased kidney), similar increases of blood pressure may occur (*lower drawing*).

renal *arteries* and *veins* conduct blood to and from the kidneys (*renal* means "involving the kidneys"). Urine empties from the kidneys into the *bladder* via the *ureters*. The bladder lies in the lower front of the *abdomen*. Urine is stored in the bladder, and when we urinate it passes out of the body through the *urethra* (Figure 3).

Approximately 25% of the blood pumped from the heart at any moment is passing through the kidneys. As a result, the entire volume of the blood in the body circulates through the kidneys every few minutes. A large proportion of this blood is processed by kidney structures called *nephrons* (Figure 4).

The nephrons are the filtering and processing factories of the kidneys. Normally people have more than one million

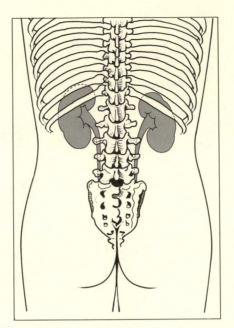

FIGURE 2
A view, from behind, of the location of the kidneys in a normal individual.

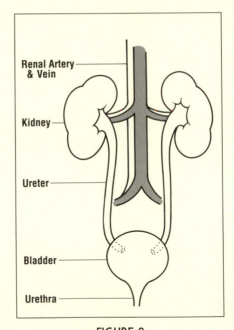

FIGURE 3
An illustration of the renal arteries and veins and the major structures of the urinary system.

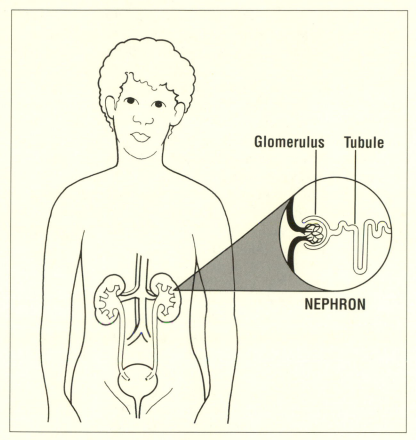

FIGURE 4
Each of the one million or so of the functioning units of the kidney, called
the nephrons, is made up of a glomerulus and a connected tubule. These
nephrons form urine from the liquid portion of the blood and transmit this
urine into the urinary drainage system.

nephrons in each kidney. Blood flows into the beginning
part of the nephron—called the *glomerulus*—where some
of the water is removed from the blood. This filtered water
contains dissolved minerals and waste products from the
blood. When this liquid passes down the long and complex
tubule, important materials can be reabsorbed back into the
bloodstream while excessive minerals and waste products

are excreted in the tubule fluid. By the time this water reaches the ureters, it has become urine. To accomplish this, normal adult kidneys process more than 60 gallons of blood a day.

The pressure in the blood vessels supplying the nephron is constantly monitored by the kidneys. This monitoring system has the ability to secrete a *hormone* named *renin*. When renin is released into the bloodstream it stimulates two major actions. The first results in the contraction of blood vessels in the body. The second causes excess salt and water to be passed from the nephron back into the bloodstream. (Note that the amount of salt—usually in the form of sodium chloride—and water in the body are closely related.) Both of these actions lead to a prompt rise in blood pressure (Figure 1).

Other hormones are produced by the kidneys. One of the most important is the active form of *vitamin D*. This vitamin is a part of an elaborate system for maintaining normal calcium balance in the body. Calcium is not only important for normal bone strength and growth, it is also essential in many of the chemical reactions constantly going on in the body. Therefore, a complex arrangement of checks and balances is necessary.

When vitamin D is ingested (such as from fortified milk), it passes into the bloodstream to the liver, where it is partly activated, and then to the kidney, where activation is completed. The active form of this vitamin can then cause the intestine to absorb more calcium from ingested food. It also can help regulate the inflow and outflow of calcium from bone. Vitamin D often works in association with *parathyroid hormone,* which is produced in small glands in the neck. Certain types of kidney disorders can cause abnormal function of both vitamin D and parathyroid hormone, resulting in serious problems with both calcium absorption and bone growth.

One other important hormone produced by the kidneys is *erythropoietin.* This hormone stimulates the *bone marrow* to produce *red blood cells,* thereby functioning as one of several systems to prevent *anemia.*

Kidney Diseases

Diseases of the kidneys are often divided into nephrologic (those that can be treated with medicine or nonsurgical treatments) and urologic (those that often require surgery). Nephrologists are doctors who specialize in providing medical treatment of kidney and *urinary tract* disorders, while urologists primarily provide surgical treatment. Children with kidney diseases, however, often require both types of treatment and therefore receive care from both types of specialists.

Another common way of labeling kidney diseases is by using several descriptive terms. *Congenital* disease refers to problems present at or shortly following birth. These problems usually arise from abnormal development of some part of the kidneys or urinary tract, or from injury to the urinary system during fetal development. These types of disorders are often distinguished from acquired diseases that may occur at any time later. *Hereditary* kidney disease refers to a predisposition in certain families to a particular type of disorder. While hereditary problems may be present at birth (congenital), they often appear later and may be undetectable for many years. A more detailed discussion of these problems can be found in chapter 3.

It is important to realize that all kidney and urinary tract diseases do not cause health problems in necessarily the same manner. For example, the type of injury that occurs in the kidney as a result of repeated infections may be very different from the type that occurs as a result of a congenital disorder.

Health Consequences of Kidney Diseases

Many diseases of the kidneys injure or affect several functioning structures. However, the original type of injury as well as its severity often determines the initial health consequences—the symptoms. For example, consider two children with poor kidney function. One child first came to his doctor's attention after developing vomiting and a severe headache that would not go away. The doctor found a very elevated blood pressure as a result of *inflammation* in the kidneys. The other youngster was found to have a similar degree of abnormal kidney function when her doctor was testing her for poor growth. Her blood pressure was normal but she was found to have a hereditary kidney problem.

Thus, various hereditary or acquired diseases may result in different types of kidney dysfunction and symptoms. Diseases that cause slow, often undetected, lessening of the kidneys' filtering ability frequently cause few symptoms. It may be years before the findings of *uremia* (kidney failure) appear. Certain other diseases that reduce kidney filtration may cause fluid retention, discolored urine, or high blood pressure.

Some diseases injure the tubules and supporting structure of the kidneys. They may occur with recurrent kidney infections or certain types of cystic diseases (see chapter 3). The initial symptoms of these diseases may include excessive urine production, abnormal blood tests, or poor growth as a result of disturbed kidney hormone production.

As you can see, the type of disease determining the symptoms often helps a doctor diagnose the problem. But some diseases affect more than one structure of the kidney. As a result, symptoms of different kidney diseases may overlap, making a clear diagnosis of the problem very difficult. Also, many of the symptoms of serious kidney problems develop slowly and may be so subtle that they remain unnoticed for a long period of time.

A summary of common symptoms of various kidney disorders appears in Table 1. Keep in mind that not all people have all symptoms. Also, many of the symptoms listed may be a result of problems elsewhere in the body. Your doctor generally can determine the presence and cause of these and other related problems through regular checkups and, if necessary, laboratory testing. A discussion of common types of health screening for kidney problems follows in the next chapter.

Table 1. Signs and symptoms that may indicate a kidney or urinary problem*

Weak or interrupted urine stream (especially in boys)
Crying or pain during urination
Recurrent unexplained fever
Foul-smelling, cloudy, or discolored urine
Low back or side pain
High blood pressure
Frequent unexplained headaches
Poor growth or bone problems
Excessive thirst
Persistent bedwetting beyond 5 years of age
Swelling (especially of face and/or feet and legs)

*Although the signs and symptoms in this table do not always mean a child has a kidney problem, it would be advisable to see your doctor if any of these appear.

Chapter 2
Is There a Kidney Problem?

We often hear patients and their family members say that doctors do too many tests. It is true that repeated physical examinations and laboratory tests can get to be a real drag. But it is important to remember that there are very good reasons for these procedures, and that they are done not just *to* the patient, but *for* the patient. Also, they provide answers to a question we often hear from the parents of our patients: "How can I be sure that my child doesn't have a kidney disease?"

Although the signs and symptoms listed in Table 1 do not always mean a child has a kidney problem, it would be advisable to see your doctor if any of these appear. Often, however, a serious problem may exist yet be "silent" for months or even years. How, then, can you be sure that a serious health problem is not being missed? This chapter explains the examinations and tests doctors can use to detect kidney disorders.

Routine Health Screening

Regular checkups by your child's physician are an important part of good health care. The current routine health care recommendations of the American Academy of Pediatrics include, among other things, periodic evaluation of growth,

13

measurement of blood pressure (beginning at age 3), testing of the blood for anemia (a low number of red blood cells,
which carry oxygen), and examination of the urine. It should
be noted that, in recent years, the benefit of routine urine
examination in the otherwise healthy child has been called
into question. In the absence of any signs or symptoms of
kidney disease, however, this system of regular examinations will greatly decrease the likelihood of missing something important.

Not too long ago, one of us saw a very pleasant, healthy-
appearing 8-year-old boy who had not been to a doctor in
a long while. When his parents finally took him to see a
pediatrician, the boy said that he often felt like his bladder
was full, even after urination. A simple physical examination
led the doctor to find a major urinary tract problem, which
could have resulted in permanent kidney failure. The problem has since been corrected, but the boy unfortunately has
been left with less than normal kidney function, which might
have been avoided by earlier detection.

Frequent Findings: Important or Not?

During a routine examination, your child's physician
may find something that might or might not be significant.
There are many such preliminary findings that lead the doctor to ask the question, "What is the likelihood that this
points to a health problem?" Often, the doctor will refer the
child to a specialist with the experience to help provide the
answer.

The three most common reasons for which we are asked
to see an otherwise healthy youngster are elevated blood
pressures (*hypertension*), very small amounts of blood in the
urine (microscopic *hematuria*), and *protein* in the urine.

Hypertension is the medical term for high blood pressure.
Over the past decade, we have become more sensitive to
the importance of childhood hypertension and its potential for long-term damaging effects. A large proportion of

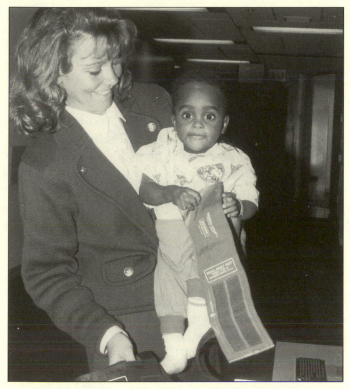

FIGURE 5
Anthony feels that it is only fair for social worker Missy Brown to get *her* blood pressure measured during *his* regular checkup.

children with hypertension will have correctable conditions, and as many as 80% of these conditions will be due to a disorder of the kidney. Therefore, a careful search for an identifiable cause for hypertension in childhood is justified (Figure 5).

A single abnormal blood pressure reading, however, does not necessarily mean a child has hypertension. The measurement of blood pressure in young children is fraught with potential problems. Erroneous readings can be caused by taking the measurement during a period of anxiety (just visiting the doctor can raise blood pressure in some children and adults), by using the wrong-sized blood pressure cuff, and by not determining the proper readings because of noise or distraction. In addition, as many as 90% of children with a high initial blood pressure measurement will be normal on later measurements.

Therefore, while a careful search for undiscovered kidney disorders is sometimes necessary in a child referred because of high blood pressure, the consultant's first task is often to determine if the child actually does have hypertension. In this way, costly, time-consuming, and potentially painful tests may be avoided.

Small amounts of blood or protein in the urine also require further investigation. Their presence in the urine will not, by themselves, cause harm. Rather, they serve as little alarms that tell the physician to check into why they are there.

Blood may appear in the urine as a result of damage to the nephrons (the main blood-filtering structures in the kidneys), urinary infection, structural abnormalities in the kidneys, or physical injury to the kidneys. Or, the blood may appear as a result of unusually vigorous activity, in which case there is probably no kidney disorder.

Proteins make up an important group of substances in the body. Therefore, the kidneys do not allow very much protein to be lost in the urine while performing their filtering jobs. The appearance of an abnormal amount of protein may signal that the normal filtering process is disrupted, possibly because damage to the kidneys is interfering with normal function. On the other hand, many children and young adults tend to excrete slightly higher amounts of protein when they exercise or stand for a long time. If this is the case, there is no increased risk of kidney disease.

Therefore, the first step in evaluating these relatively common findings is to identify which children have harmless findings and which children require a more careful evaluation. This process often is not as easy as it may sound. Sometimes a pediatric nephrologist or urologist is asked to assist in this determination.

Common Evaluations of the Kidneys and Urinary Tract

Many different types of tests may be used in an attempt to identify the presence and nature of disorders of the kidneys and urinary tract. Parents and older children often are confused by the need for so many tests and by discussions of the information they provide. As we describe some of the more common tests, remember that there are many types of tests that can answer the same question equally well. Your doctor may decide to use certain tests based on their availability and his or her clinical experience.

Blood and Urine Tests

Creatinine is often used as a measurement of overall kidney function. The substance creatinine is a waste product of the muscles. It is filtered out of the blood by the kidneys. Since the amount of muscle tissue in our bodies changes little from day to day, the production of creatinine remains fairly constant. Therefore, we can estimate the efficiency of kidney function by measuring the amount of creatinine in the blood. A somewhat more accurate estimate of kidney function can be made by measuring the level of creatinine in a timed urine collection (discussed on p. 18), which may be done at the same time as the blood test.

Urea nitrogen measurement is similar to that of creatinine in that it provides information about an individual's kidney function (i.e., ability to excrete waste products). The measurement is often referred to as either the blood urea nitrogen (*BUN*) or serum urea nitrogen (*SUN*). Urea nitrogen differs from creatinine in that it is produced by the body as a result of the "burning" of proteins for energy. Because it is excreted by the kidney in a somewhat different manner than creatinine, its measurement in the blood provides additional information. The measurement of both urea nitrogen and creatinine provides information not only about kidney function, but about the child's state of *hydration* and diet as well.

Kidney disease or its treatment can result in abnormal concentrations of minerals and other compounds, which may harm many important body functions. The most common of these substances that doctors test for in the blood are sodium, potassium, chloride, and carbon dioxide (collectively referred to as the *electrolytes*), and calcium, phosphorus, and magnesium.

Another important test is the complete blood count (CBC). It provides information about the different types of blood cells, including the amount of red blood cells. This test is obtained frequently in children with advanced kidney disease, because anemia is common in these children and may contribute to fatigue. *White blood cells* (which help fight infection) and *platelets* (which assist in blood clotting) are also measured in the CBC.

The timed collection of urine often is used by doctors to study certain useful aspects of kidney function. A specimen is most commonly collected over a 24-hour period. Frequently, children and parents fail to collect timed urine specimens completely or properly (see below). Errors lead to incorrect or uninterpretable results and much frustration and wasted time. This test can be very useful, however, if a few simple directions are followed. When the collection period begins (usually in the morning), the child should urinate and discard the urine. This empties the bladder in preparation for the timed collection. Following this, all urine should be added to the collection container until the child voids one last time, which should be 24 hours after the collection began. This final voiding should be added to the collection container and the time noted. Since urinating is such an automatic process for most of us, we find that at some point during the collection period, children and even adolescents may forget to collect their urine. Therefore, it helps for parents to remind children frequently in order to avoid having to collect the urine a second time. Finally, to minimize odor and the growth of bacteria, the container should be placed in a paper bag and kept in a cool place.

Radiology Studies

There are many tests of the kidneys and bladder that can be done by a radiologist. This doctor is usually thought of as the X-ray specialist, but there are actually many imaging tests that do not use X rays. Many parents of growing children are concerned about their child's exposure to X rays during the many tests performed during a kidney disease evaluation. Although it is a good idea to avoid unnecessary radiation exposure, the actual amount of exposure from commonly used tests is relatively small. It may be reassuring to compare radiation exposure from X rays to the exposure we get each day from natural sources (the earth, sun, and space). For example, a routine X ray of the chest exposes the child to an amount of radiation equal to the natural radiation exposure occurring in approximately one week. Different studies require different exposures and numbers of pictures, and hence the amount of radiation will vary. If you still feel your child is being overexposed to X rays, discuss this with the radiologist or with your doctor.

Radiologic tests of the kidneys and bladder fall into two general categories: tests that tell us something about the structure of the kidneys and urinary tract, and tests that give information about certain aspects of their function. The specific tests performed will depend upon the type of problem being evaluated. The more commonly used tests use either sound waves (*ultrasound*), conventional X rays (*radiology*), or very small amounts of radioactive materials (*nuclear medicine*) to obtain the necessary information. Figure 6 compares the pictures obtained from three commonly used radiologic studies of the kidneys. A brief description of the more common tests follows.

In situations where it is not necessary to obtain the most detailed picture of the kidneys, ultrasonography is often used. This technique employs harmless, high-frequency sound waves (ultrasound) that cannot be heard by the human ear. Much in the same way that a submarine takes a "picture" of the ocean bottom with sonar, the sonogram provides a view of the kidneys and surrounding structures. This

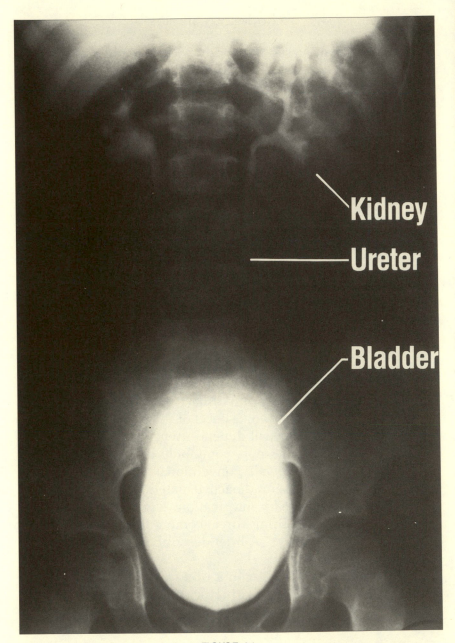

FIGURE 6A
Three of the more common types of radiographic studies of the kidney. Figure 6A uses conventional X rays to obtain an intravenous pyelogram (IVP). The major structures of the urinary drainage system may be accurately discerned by this type of test.

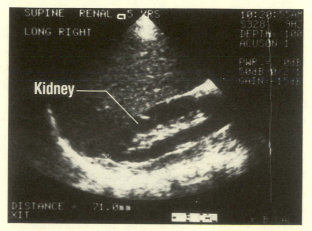

FIGURE 6B

Figure 6B demonstrates the appearance of the kidney using sound waves, rather than conventional X rays. Although the structures are not as well demonstrated by this test, as compared to the IVP, experienced radiologists can extract a great deal of structural information from the sonogram while avoiding the need for exposure to X rays or injected materials.

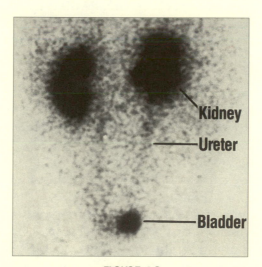

FIGURE 6C

Figure 6C shows one type of renal scan, which uses minute quantities of special radioisotopes. Compared to the two examples above, the renal scan generally gives less *structural* information about the urinary system, while providing information about certain *functional* aspects of the kidneys and urinary system.

test is often selected as a first study because it is considered safe, is completely painless, and provides a good deal of information.

The excretory urogram (also called the intravenous pyelogram or IVP) is an X-ray study that requires the intravenous injection of a material that is then excreted by the kidneys. This study generally provides excellent pictures of the structure of the kidneys and the entire urinary system. However, the results may be less satisfactory in very small children. In addition, a very small number of children may be allergic to the injected material. Although the detailed information provided by this test is valuable, many physicians prefer other tests that avoid exposure to X rays and potential allergic reactions.

Another X-ray test sometimes used for greater structural detail is the computerized tomogram (CT or CAT scan). The CT scanner can take X-ray pictures of the urinary system from many different angles. Then the computer assembles the X rays into a cross-sectional image that can be studied for structural abnormalities.

Radiologists in a specialty called nuclear medicine have developed several imaging compounds that are excreted by the kidneys in a variety of ways. These compounds are "labeled" with very small amounts of radioactive material and are then injected into a vein. As they pass through the kidneys, a sensitive camera that detects the radioactivity records their trail. Often called *renal* scans, these studies have become extremely valuable tests of different aspects of kidney function. They expose a child to about the same amount of radiation as the IVP or less.

Often, radiologic studies of the bladder and lower urinary tract are necessary. The most commonly used test is the voiding cystourethrogram (or VCUG), which is a complicated term for a picture of the bladder and urethra. This test requires placing a *catheter* through the urethra and into the bladder. A material similar to that used in the IVP is then placed in the bladder through the catheter, and X-ray pictures are taken before and during voiding. Since this material is not injected into the bloodstream, there is little risk of an allergic reaction. It is the insertion of the catheter that most often takes persuasion and a gentle touch. Under certain circumstances, a radionuclide cystogram can be used as an alternative to the VCUG. This technique also requires a catheter, but it uses a material to view the bladder that is similar to that used in the renal scan. Although this test does not provide as much detail as a VCUG, it exposes the child to considerably less radiation.

Kidney Biopsy

There are times when, despite obtaining many blood, urine, and radiologic tests, the nephrologist is still not certain about the type or extent of a kidney problem, or even whether a significant one exists. Under these circumstances, a kidney *biopsy* may become necessary. For most people, a biopsy is thought of as a means for diagnosing cancer. Cancer of the kidney in children is rather rare and is usually diagnosed by other tests. When a pediatric nephrologist suggests a kidney biopsy, he or she is referring to the removal of a small piece of kidney tissue for examination under the microscope. When interpreted together with other tests, the biopsy often results in a specific diagnosis. It also can give the nephrologist information about the activity or extent of a disease process, which is valuable in making treatment decisions.

Today virtually all kidney biopsies are done by placing a special biopsy needle through the skin and muscles of the back into the kidney. There are rare occasions when a formal operation is still necessary. Each physician who performs biopsies may do so a little differently. Therefore, although we will give a general description of the procedure, the details may vary from doctor to doctor.

Most physicians will obtain a radiologic study of the kidneys prior to the biopsy. Some use the IVP or a similar procedure; some use the sonogram. The patient frequently will receive a sedative before the biopsy; sometimes a patient must be put to sleep. The patient will be placed on a firm ta-

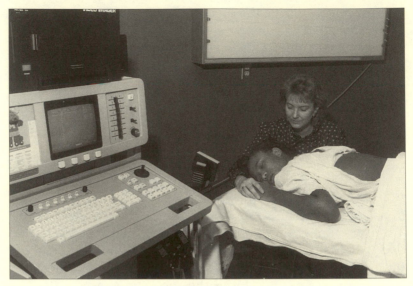

FIGURE 7

This young lady, accompanied by nurse practitioner Betsy Nicolli, has received a mild sedative and has been placed in position for her renal biopsy. The ultrasound machine, which is used to obtain the renal sonogram, can be seen on the left.

ble, sometimes with a roll of towels under the belly (see Figure 7). Under sterile procedures, the skin is numbed with a local anesthetic, and the biopsy needle is then inserted into the kidney. This needle allows the withdrawal of a small piece of kidney tissue, generally about 1/2 to 3/4 of an inch long and about the thickness of a spaghetti noodle. Following the procedure, the patient is usually returned to the hospital room to rest for a day or two. It is common for the urine to appear bloody for a short time following a biopsy. If this occurs, don't panic; just promptly inform the nurse.

Perhaps the experience of undergoing a kidney biopsy is best explained by a patient who has had one (see Figure 8):

"My name is Erica and I am a 16-year-old kidney patient at Children's Hospital. My biopsy was not a horrible or terrifying

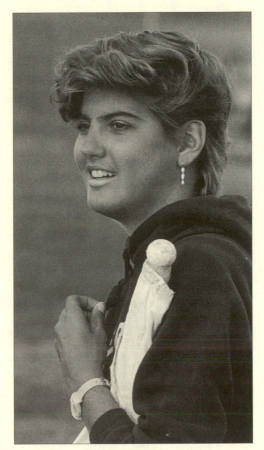

FIGURE 8
Erica tells of her kidney biopsy experience.

experience. In fact, the worst part was having to stay in bed and being forced to use a bedpan. I was under a sedative during the whole procedure and really couldn't have cared less. I was given a local anesthetic with a needle to numb my skin; this pinched and stung a bit. After that, I couldn't feel the biopsy needle except for a slight pressure. When the actual sample was taken, I felt as though the breath had been knocked out of me a little bit. It wasn't painful, just unpleasant, and very brief. Looking back, I feel that the procedure was simple and not very painful."

Erica's mother added an interesting comment that we have heard many times before. She felt Erica's biggest problem before the biopsy was her anxiety:

"Although Erica was told what might hurt and what probably wouldn't, she worried that the doctors weren't telling her everything and that the biopsy would be more painful than it actually was."

It is important to understand why a biopsy is being done on your child and what information it might provide. Issues to discuss with your doctor include the use of sedative medication (mild sedatives are often used; general anesthesia is less common) and the type of activity restriction required following the procedure. With modern technology, the risks involved in kidney biopsy are very small. It is not unusual for there to be visible blood in the urine after kidney biopsy. Occasionally, there may be bleeding around the kidney that causes abdominal or back pain. Your doctor will discuss the risks involved in kidney biopsy at the time consent for the procedure is obtained.

Making the Diagnosis

Parents and children naturally have questions during examinations and procedures, and they are encouraged to ask them. Questions about the test results and the diagnosis are best answered by the specialist or the patient's primary doctor, after all testing has been completed. Most of the other doctors, nurses, and radiologic technicians the family may encounter will provide information about a specific procedure or test, but they often will not discuss the results or speculate about the diagnosis. This is not because they want to hide anything from the patient or family, but because they only have pieces of the total information that goes into making an accurate diagnosis.

After the scheduled examinations and tests are completed and the doctor has had time to go over the results, a meeting often is held with the family to discuss whether anything abnormal has been found. It is very important at this meeting to ask any questions you might have. Also, if you don't understand something the doctor says, ask for an explanation in simpler terms. And, if you think of any questions later, feel free to contact the doctor to discuss them.

Sometimes it is not possible to reach a clear diagnosis right away. It may be necessary to do more tests or to wait for a period of time to see whether the symptoms change or to evaluate the response to specific medications. The family can help greatly by staying in touch with the doctor to report any changes, especially worsening of the symptoms.

If a kidney disorder is diagnosed, the doctor will discuss whatever steps seem most necessary to treat the problem or possibly several options. Again, this is an important time for parents and older children to ask any questions they might have about the diagnosis. Sometimes, especially if surgery is suggested or the problem is thought to be quite severe, families might want to get a second opinion (see chapter 10). This will often reassure the family that the steps being taken are the most prudent ones.

Chapter 3
Congenital, Hereditary, and Acquired Kidney Diseases

Many of the diseases of the kidney discussed in this chapter are serious ones, often leading to significant and possibly permanent health problems. Certainly, having a child with such problems is of great concern to the family. However, the explosion of medical progress that has been made in the recognition and treatment of many of these diseases is very encouraging. We hope that some understanding of how a child develops a particular kidney problem, coupled with knowledge of the progress that has been made, will give parents reason to be realistic yet optimistic about their child's future.

There are too many types of specific kidney disorders to describe in detail in this book. However, it is useful to present information on the basic origins and consequences of three general types of diseases. In chapter 1 we introduced these three types: congenital, hereditary, and acquired kidney disease. In this chapter we will go a step further, to discuss how each type of kidney disease occurs and the problems it causes.

In understanding how kidney diseases develop, it may help to compare the disease process to the building of a dam across a swiftly flowing river (Figure 9). In order to have a perfectly functioning dam (assuming we were qualified dam builders), we would need a good design, and strong bricks and mortar used precisely according to the design. Furthermore, we would have to hope that good weather would be

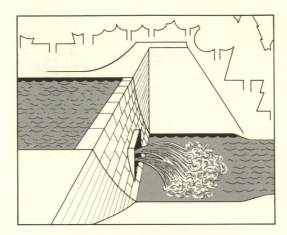

FIGURE 9

A properly built dam requires a good plan and strong materials in addition to careful construction. Similarly, the genetic plan for formation of the kidneys must include a correct design as well as the use, by the body, of normally formed construction materials.

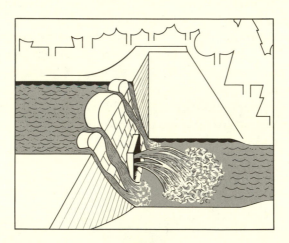

FIGURE 10

Sometimes, there is interference with the normal development of the kidneys. Often, this results in an abnormality of the structure of the kidneys or some part of the urinary system. When this occurs, the kidneys may be unable to perform all of their normal functions, much like this abnormally constructed dam cannot hold back water in the way that was originally intended.

on our side during the building and that no extreme floods would damage the dam. Applying this analogy to the urinary system and kidneys, think of the design as heredity, the construction process as the development that occurs during pregnancy, and the weather as the various environmental factors that can harm the kidneys.

Congenital Kidney Disease

The first signs of kidney development in the fetus can be found as early as the first month of pregnancy, although permanent kidney formation does not begin until about one month later. The normal development of the kidneys goes through several stages, with four totally separate structures growing and developing: kidneys, ureters, bladder, and urethra. The development of the urinary system also is closely associated with genital development. By the time this development process is completed at the end of pregnancy, more than one million individual nephrons are formed in each kidney and connected to the drainage and storage system of the kidneys (the ureters, bladder, and urethra). No new nephrons are formed after birth.

This process is so complex and orderly, it is a wonder that it succeeds so often. When this development does not proceed properly, major abnormalities of the kidneys or lower urinary system, including the genitals, may occur. These problems are akin to a major construction mistake in our dam-building project (Figure 10). Even perfect materials won't make a good dam if the dam isn't put together right in the first place.

The most important congenital problems that occur are (1) complete failure of kidney formation, (2) abnormal nephron formation, and (3) problems with the drainage of urine.

Complete failure of formation of kidneys is called *aplasia*. If only one kidney is absent and the other is normal, a normal lifespan can be expected. Aplasia of both kidneys is associated with diminished amniotic fluid, and newborns with this problem often have severe lung disease leading to death. This occurs because normal lung development depends on the formation of amniotic fluid by the fetal kidneys. When kidney formation occurs, but there is improper nephron formation, this may result in fewer nephrons than expected (*hypoplasia*) or in undeveloped, poorly functioning nephrons (*dysplasia*). Dysplasia is often associated with fluid-filled *cysts* in the kidneys (*cystic dysplasia*).

Since the extent of these abnormalities varies from mild to severe, so does the degree of kidney disease they cause. A moderate abnormality may give the infant enough kidney function to thrive normally, but it can lead to progressive worsening of kidney function or even kidney failure after months or years. Poor kidney function may include problems with holding on to body water efficiently (which can cause dehydration when the infant is sick, for instance, with diarrhea) and in maintaining normal chemical balance in the body.

Finally, problems with drainage of the urine take on many forms. There may be partial or complete blockage of urine out of one or both kidneys in any of the places shown in Figure 11. This blockage causes pressure to build up in the kidney while interfering with the normal excretion of urine. With this pressure buildup, damage to kidney tissue can occur, both on a microscopic level in the nephrons and visibly as shown in the figure. If the blockage of urine is severe enough, or remains undetected long enough, the kidney damage can be permanent and may lead to the same type of progressive problems as does dysplasia.

Two special forms of urine drainage problems include *reflux* and the prune belly syndrome. In reflux (discussed in more detail in chapter 4), urine may freely flow backward into the kidney from the bladder. When this is severe, and particularly in association with infection in the urinary system, severe kidney damage occurs. Children with the prune belly syndrome have multiple abnormalities of the urinary tract, often with poorly draining and enlarged ureters, dysplasia, and frequent other structural abnormalities. Its name comes from the wrinkled appearance of the abdominal wall due to

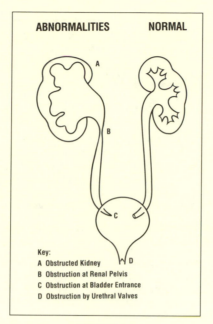

ABNORMALITIES   NORMAL

Key:
A Obstructed Kidney
B Obstruction at Renal Pelvis
C Obstruction at Bladder Entrance
D Obstruction by Urethral Valves

FIGURE 11
This drawing shows the major sites of potential obstruction to urine flow
within the urinary system.

underdevelopment of the abdominal muscles. It most often
occurs in males and is usually accompanied by undescended
testes.

Hereditary Kidney Disease

Let's return to our dam-building project. Your engineer may
have carried out the design instructions perfectly. If there
was a mistake or hidden flaw in the design, however, the
quality of your dam would suffer from an imperfect structure
that could weaken over time (Figure 12). This is a problem
similar to many hereditary diseases of the kidneys.

Hereditary (or genetic) disease, in general, refers to certain
characteristics of the body that are transmitted from a parent

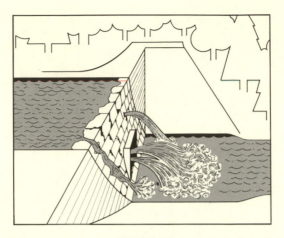

FIGURE 12
Although some of the hereditary problems affecting the kidneys may be evident early in life, many can be quite subtle in the young child. Similarly, a properly constructed dam, made with inferior materials, may begin to deteriorate earlier than expected.

to children. This process of inheritance is extremely complex, and it often does not occur in a straightforward manner. For example, eye color is inherited. Brown-eyed parents are more likely to have a brown-eyed child; they may, however, have one with blue eyes. This is because the parents may carry the genes for both brown and blue eyes, and therefore have the capacity to transfer the blue color to their son or daughter. In much this same way, inherited abnormalities of the kidneys may be transferred to children even if the parents have no significant abnormalities of their own kidneys.

To further confuse the situation, some hereditary problems may only mildly affect one family member and thus remain undetected, while another has a serious problem. Finally, since these hereditary disorders may come from subtle gene abnormalities, they may not even have been detected in previous generations. Perhaps the person with the disorder did not live long enough for a serious problem to appear, or maybe the disorder was not severe enough to cause the person to seek treatment.

The occurrence of a hereditary problem in a child often causes a dilemma for parents who are considering having more children. For this reason, we recommend that these families arrange for a consultation with a genetic specialist, who can advise families about the possible risks of having other children with similar problems.

In a sense, hereditary abnormalities are also congenital, in that they are present at birth. However, hereditary diseases often do not become evident until later in life, in much the same way that a design flaw in a dam may not lead to any detectable weakening of the dam until well after it has been built.

Among the more common inherited kidney disorders are the cystic diseases. The presence of cysts in the kidneys does not always indicate the presence of a disease that will cause health problems. Also, there are a number of cystic diseases that may be associated with other organ abnormalities. Of the inherited cystic diseases, polycystic kidney disease and medullary cystic disease are significant potential health problems.

Infantile polycystic kidney disease was the term once used to describe the cystic disease of the kidney thought to be most common in young children. Since this disorder does not exclusively occur in infants, and with better understanding of the inheritance of this disorder, it is now referred to as autosomal recessive polycystic disease. The term "autosomal recessive" refers to the fact that the inheritance factor must come from both parents in order to cause disease, and that the parents are generally unaffected—they are carriers. When the disease occurs early in life, the kidneys are commonly huge and function poorly. In fact, if the disease occurs during fetal development, the kidneys may be sufficiently large and poorly functional to interfere with normal lung development, leading to serious breathing problems at birth similar to those described for infants with aplasia. Scars may also occur in the liver in this disorder. For reasons that are poorly understood, when the disease occurs early in life, the kidney disease is severe, often leading to kidney failure (see chapter 5), while the liver involvement is minimal. There tends to be milder kidney involvement with more severe liver complications when the disease occurs in the older child and adolescent.

The other major form of polycystic kidney disease is known as autosomal dominant polycystic kidney disease. This was formerly termed adult-type polycystic disease, but it can occur in children. The term "autosomal dominant" means that inheritance from only one parent is necessary. There may be tremendous variability in the extent of the cystic abnormalities in other family members, and it is common for there to be no known other members of the family affected. This may be a result of the disease being sufficiently mild in relatives to have escaped detection, or because the disease (and the gene abnormality) has not previously existed in other family members. Children with this type of cystic disease may have very slow but progressive loss of kidney function, such that significant medical problems do not occur until well into adulthood. The disease is often diagnosed after discovery of enlarged kidneys, hypertension, or blood or protein in the urine during a physical examination. It may be found during screening evaluations of the relatives of someone found to have the disease. There is often an associated problem with efficient concentration of the urine. In addition, cysts may occur in other organs, including the liver, pancreas, lung, ovary, and certain brain blood vessels. Genetic counseling is of great importance for these children and families since there is a high risk of the disease occurring in other offspring.

Medullary cystic disease, also called by the unpronounceable term "juvenile nephronophthisis," is a disorder occurring more commonly in older children and adults. It causes progressive kidney dysfunction and often leads to kidney failure (see chapter 5). The inheritance in younger children is more likely to be autosomal recessive, similar to recessive polycystic kidney disease. When occurring in childhood, it may be associated with eye abnormalities as well as abnormalities of the liver, bone, and the nervous system. Although the early phases of progressive damage to the kidneys may be silent, many children will have excessive thirst and urination (from excreting dilute urine), anemia, or growth abnormalities that first bring them to medical attention.

Several other inherited disorders of the kidney are worthy of mention. These problems are often not as obvious as the cystic diseases but may be of equal importance. In other words, although the design of the dam may be perfect, perhaps the design of the materials used to construct it was weak. As a result, it might have minor flaws in materials that lead to leaks in the dam, or it may have major structural flaws that lead to complete collapse. Similarly, more subtle abnormalities in either kidney structure or function can result in problems that can be minimal or quite severe.

Abnormalities of the filtering *membrane* of the glomerulus may be inherited, as well. A disorder generally referred to as benign familial hematuria is one example of this type of disorder. Here, there is an abnormality in the way the filtering membrane is formed. When seen under the microscope, the membrane appears abnormally thin. Most children who are found to have this disorder first come to the physician's attention because of blood in the urine. The blood may be visible or detectable only under the microscope. An evaluation of other family members frequently reveals similar findings in a parent or sibling. In many of these children the presence of this abnormality, while undoubtedly inherited, does not cause any significant kidney dysfunction. The problem is distinguishing these youngsters from those with more serious underlying abnormalities.

The term hereditary *nephritis* denotes the presence of another abnormality of this same filtering membrane. In this case, however, the problem is more severe and may cause progressive damage to the kidneys. Recent research has shown that there are different ways this disease can be inherited. In some cases, there is a strong association with visual and/or hearing problems. This particular relationship in individuals with hereditary nephritis is called Alport syndrome.

Other abnormalities that are sometimes inherited and may cause disorders associated with the kidneys include excessive calcium excretion with a predisposition to bloody urine and/or kidney stones, sickle cell disease, functional disorders where the kidney fails to correctly regulate the formation or excretion of specific materials, and certain inflammatory diseases that are prevalent in some families and may cause inflammatory kidney diseases (see acquired kidney diseases). There are also several biochemical disorders that lead to abnormal deposits of various materials in the kidneys with resultant damage.

The manner in which hereditary abnormalities occur and their potential consequences are beyond the scope of this book. However, using your newly gained knowledge of how and why the kidney performs its assigned tasks, you are now well prepared to discuss these with your doctor.

Acquired Kidney Diseases

The design was right, the materials used were solid, and construction was properly carried out. The dam, which rose high above the river, was everyone's pride and joy. When an earthquake caused a big crack in the face of the dam, however, everyone realized that it shouldn't have been built on the San Andreas fault (Figure 13). Likewise, even perfectly formed and functioning kidneys may suffer unexpected damage. Although this type of damage may occur in many different ways, the problems that result all fall under the category of acquired disorders.

The most common acquired disease of the kidney and urinary tract is that of urinary infection. Under certain conditions, urinary infections can cause recurring and potentially serious medical problems. These are discussed separately in chapter 4.

Other acquired diseases of the kidney can be further subdivided into glomerular and tubulointerstitial diseases

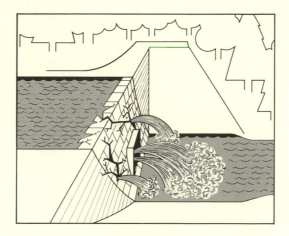

FIGURE 13
Even when everything comes out right, unexpected illness can injure the kidneys, just like our dam suffers from the unexpected earthquake.

(see chapter 1). This classification gives a better understanding of the results of these diseases, which are often quite different.

Nephritis

One type of glomerular disease is generally referred to as *glomerulonephritis,* or simply nephritis. This type of disease was formerly called Bright's disease. The "-itis" part of the term nephritis denotes inflammation. The body has several very powerful ways of causing inflammation, which is the body's reaction to injury. A small cut in the skin that becomes infected, for instance, will develop swelling, redness, and increasing tenderness. These reactions are the result of the body mobilizing its systems for fighting the infection. Certain chemical materials and blood cells produced in the body as part of the *immune system* will be deposited in the infected area to kill the invading germs as quickly as possible. If these systems did not exist we would be at the mercy of any virus or bacteria that entered the body and started multiplying.

Unfortunately, there are unusual situations when the kidney is injured as an "innocent bystander." In this situation, the immune system is directed elsewhere, but since the glomerulus of the nephron filters many substances in the blood, materials that provoke inflammation build up in the nephrons, causing nephritis. Nephritis may occur as part of certain inflammatory diseases involving other areas of the body. In other circumstances, the inflammation may be limited to the kidney. The inflammation may be short-lived, with no long-term consequences, such as those that usually occur in the nephritis that may follow certain types of strep infections. Alternatively, the inflammation may be chronic, lasting months or even years. Even after many years of study, the origin of many forms of nephritis is still unknown. Although nephritis in childhood is uncommon, it constitutes a significant group of disorders from the standpoint of kidney disease.

The symptoms and signs that arise as a consequence of nephritis are a result of the degree and duration of injury to the glomerulus. Certain signs and symptoms tend to predominate in certain diseases. Microscopic or visible blood in the urine occurs commonly. When the blood is visible, the urine is often "tea" or "cola" colored, although it can also be the color of blood. Other common abnormalities include swelling of the hands, feet, or eyes, mild or severe protein loss in the urine, hypertension, or pain in the sides over the kidneys. Rapidly or slowly progressive kidney dysfunction may occur.

The treatment of different forms of nephritis varies according to the type of disease, its severity, and the opinion of the treating physician. Treatments may be directed toward correction of associated abnormalities, such as control of hypertension if present, or correction of chemical imbalances using various medications and diets (see chapter 9). If the kidney dysfunction is sufficiently severe, even if short-lived, artificial kidney treatments (*dialysis*) may be necessary (see chapter 6). Although many forms of nephritis still have no known cure, several types may be controlled or cured using potent medications that can alter the function of the immune system. Chapter 8 contains a more detailed discussion of many of these medications.

Nephrotic syndromes

When the amount of protein lost in the urine is severe, the *nephrotic syndrome* may occur. While the body can manufacture proteins to keep up with mild to moderate protein losses in the urine, the result of massive losses in the urine is a lowering of protein levels in the blood. Proteins perform many functions in the body. One of them is to maintain the balance of water in the bloodstream. When the level of protein in the blood becomes excessively low, water will leak out into body tissue and tend to accumulate under the skin. This can result in extensive swelling (*edema*), most typically in the face, legs, and feet, and sometimes in the abdominal cavity.

During periods of swelling with the nephrotic syndrome, the kidneys may detect the diminished volume of the blood. They often attempt to adjust the abnormality by retaining salt and water. If a child with nephrotic syndrome ingests excessive amounts of salt and water during periods of edema, the amount of swelling may worsen significantly. In situations where the protein leak stops or is controlled, the swelling disappears as the water is redistributed to its proper place.

There are two common ways in which nephrotic syndrome occurs. Suppose you place some dirty garden peas in a colander, as in Figure 14A. Running water over the peas will wash out the dirt, leaving the peas behind. The glomerulus can be thought of as the colander, the peas as protein, and the dirt as the filtered waste products. In Figure 14B, the neighbor's 3-year-old has attacked your colander with a screwdriver and enlarged some of the holes. When the next batch of peas is washed, some of them will come out through the bigger holes and be lost down the drain. This is an example of how progressive damage to the glomerulus can result

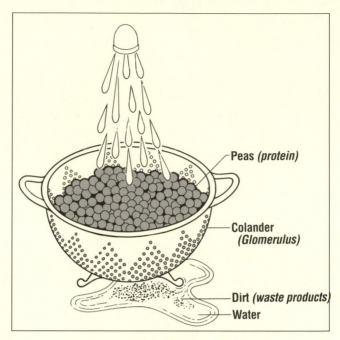

FIGURE 14A
Normally, the kidneys can filter impurities from the blood, while conserving important materials such as proteins. This is similar to the process whereby a kitchen colander can use running water (the urine) to remove dirt (body waste) without losing the peas (proteins) down the drain.

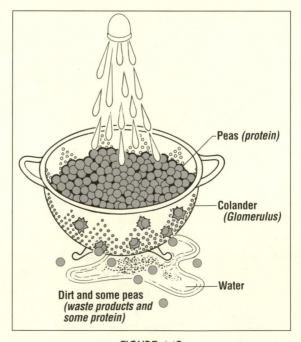

FIGURE 14B
Physical damage to the walls of the colander can allow some of the peas to run out, much in the same way that microscopic damage to the filtering surface of the glomerulus can cause protein to be lost in the urine.

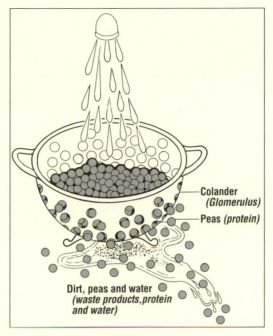

Colander
(Glomerulus)

Peas (protein)

Dirt, peas and water
(waste products, protein
and water)

FIGURE 14C

In certain forms of nephrotic syndrome, protein is lost in the urine when the filter loses its ability to "screen" filtered substances properly. This is as if the colander you normally use suddenly had each one of its holes stretched to a size that was larger than the peas you were washing. Naturally, the peas would pass through and down the drain in great numbers.

in an increasing amount of protein loss into the urine, such as occurs with nephritis.

The other form of acquired nephrotic syndrome that occursin childhood is the most common type. It has been called by several different names, including *nil disease, minimal change disease,* and *lipoid nephrosis,* among others. This form is not associated with nephritis. To use the previous example, rather than the colander's being attacked by a screwdriver, imagine that its holes suddenly got much bigger, as in Figure 14C. Now the peas can flow freely down the drain along with the dirt and water. In this form of nephrotic syndrome, filtration in the glomerulus is drastically altered so that substances, such as proteins, are excreted into the urine. This most often occurs in young children, and it is characterized by the rather sudden onset of episodes of swelling associated with urine protein loss, frequently following an otherwise minor illness.

It is common for the first episode of nephrotic syndrome to be initially thought of as an "allergic reaction." This is because of the common occurrence of relapse of the disease with a "cold" and the frequent observation of facial swelling. The facial swelling, like all of the other fluid accumulation of the nephrotic syndrome, is transient and will resolve when the disease relapse is controlled.

In addition to swelling, children with minimal change disease are, among other things, at increased risk for more serious infections during the episodes of swelling, since some of the proteins that are lost in the urine are important to the immune system. The majority of cases of this form of nephrotic syndrome can be controlled with medications, most commonly steroids (see chapter 9). Steroids do not cure the disease but often very effectively control it. Nonetheless, many of the affected children will have recurring episodes of swelling that may continue throughout childhood. This does not necessarily mean that the disease is progressing. Rather, it means that the disease has not yet resolved; it will eventually disappear in most children.

One of the major treatment problems in children with medication (steroid)-controlled nephrotic syndrome who have frequent relapses is the cumulative side effects of the steroid medication (see chapter 9). In fact, one of the challenges to the pediatric nephrologist is the construction of a treatment program that will adequately control the disease while minimizing toxicity of the medication. Although this is not always possible, children with frequently relapsing nephrotic syndrome who are developing serious side effects from steroids can be considered for alternative forms of therapy, including use of the drugs cyclophosphamide, chlorambucil, or cyclosporine A (see chapter 9). There is, unfortunately, a small percentage of children with the nephrotic syndrome who fail to respond to medical treatment. Many of these children eventually develop damage to the kidneys and, ultimately, kidney failure.

Hemolytic-Uremic Syndrome

One final glomerular disease that is worthy of separate mention is the *hemolytic-uremic syndrome*. This disease most commonly occurs following a diarrheal or respiratory illness in young children. It is usually characterized by sudden and severe kidney failure associated with the formation of clots in the small blood vessels of the kidney and the breakdown of red blood cells, which can lead to severe anemia. Hypertension, often also severe, frequently occurs as well. There may be associated neurologic problems and intestinal bleeding. Although several experimental treatments for this disease have been investigated, there is not yet any conclusive evidence that they are beneficial in all patients. Fortunately, however, most episodes of this disease resolve spontaneously over several days or weeks, and kidney function frequently returns to normal. Therefore, the mainstay of therapy for hemolytic-uremic syndrome is to prevent any life-threatening complication of the kidney failure, such as hypertension, anemia, and clotting disturbances, while the disease runs its course. This supportive treatment often requires some form of dialysis, since the kidney failure may last days or weeks or, rarely, longer. With the liberal use of dialysis as supportive treatment, there has been a remarkable improvement of ultimate outcome in terms of survival and recovery of kidney function.

The final group of acquired kidney diseases to consider are the tubulointerstitial disorders. This term refers to diseases that cause inflammation or injury to the tissue surrounding the nephrons (the interstitium) and the kidney tubules. These disorders may be rather sudden and severe or chronic, and generally result from injury to the kidney tubules caused by a chemical or unusual side effect of certain medications, or from an inflammatory process similar to that which occurs in glomerulonephritis.

The kidney tubules and interstitium seem to be particularly sensitive to injury from a variety of substances. These include certain antibiotics, other drugs (including many over-the-counter pain medications), certain ingested toxic materials (for example, lead, mercury, and antifreeze, among many others), underlying biochemical disturbances in the body, and a variety of infections.

In adults, tubulointerstitial disease is a major cause of kidney failure, commonly associated with chronic use of various analgesics. In children, tubulointerstitial disease is much less common. In situations where kidney damage occurs from ingestion of a toxic material or as a result of inflammation from the ingestion of a particular drug, further damage may be avoided by prompt treatment. Unfortunately, in many circumstances the disease has been present for some time before symptoms appear, and the material causing the damage remains undiscovered. This can result in permanent or progressive kidney disease.

Although tubulointerstitial disease may be discovered during the investigation of blood or protein in the urine, or of abnormal growth, it is often silently progressive. In the early phases of the disease, hypertension and edema are uncommon, but there may be frequent chemical abnormalities in the body as a result of disturbed function of the kidney tubules.

About Your Child

With this information on the three general categories of kidney disorders, you should be able to understand how your child's disease developed. If you have questions about the specific type of disease affecting your child, discuss this with your doctor. With this basic information about your child's disease, you may be better able to accept it and become involved in obtaining the best possible treatment. You will also be better able to help your child understand, cope with, and adjust to whatever stresses are related to the disease.

Chapter 4
Urinary Tract Infections in Children

(Authors' note: Dr. H. Guilford Rushton, Vice Chairman of Pediatric Urology at Children's National Medical Center, coauthored this chapter.)

Infection of the urinary system, or "urinary tract," is one of the most common bacterial infections occurring in children. Urinary infections can become a significant medical problem if not treated promptly and adequately, and they can lead to serious complications. Most of the common infections of the urinary tract are caused by bacterial germs. When the infection is limited to the bladder, this is called *cystitis*. A more serious infection involving the kidney is referred to as *pyelonephritis*.

These two types of infection differ not only in the symptoms they produce, but also in the potential long-term consequences they may cause. Cystitis is generally a milder illness, whereas even a single episode of pyelonephritis, particularly in infants and toddlers, may cause permanent damage to the kidneys.

Causes of Urinary Tract Infections

Urinary tract infections are generally caused by bacteria that invade the urinary tract. These infections are not contagious to others. In most cases, the bacteria enter the urinary system by passing up the urethra into the bladder.

Therefore, the most common types of bacteria causing urinary infections are those that usually live on the skin near

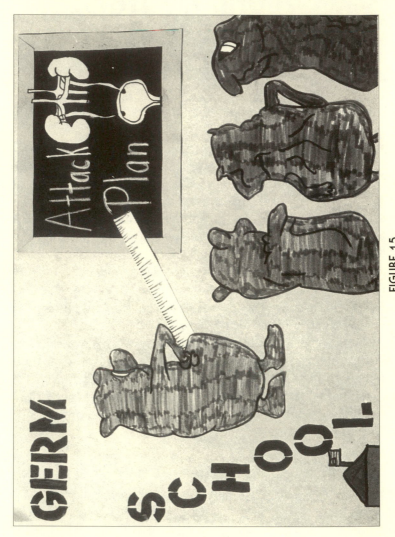

FIGURE 15

An entry in the National Gift of Life Poster and Essay Contest.

the opening of the urethra. These include common skin bacterial germs as well as those that come from the child's intestinal tract (rectum). Unfortunately, no reasonable amount of good skin hygiene can completely eradicate these bacteria.

Except during infancy, urinary infections occur about three times more commonly in girls than in boys. This is partly because the urethra of a girl is much shorter than that of a boy, providing easier passage of bacteria into the bladder. Also, in girls the opening of the urethra is close to the vagina, where bacteria normally grow.

Some people with urinary infection appear to have a lower resistance to the bacteria commonly found on the skin near the opening of the urethra. The reason for this is not completely understood, but it seems to be a problem that occurs in many children who are prone to infections of the urinary tract. Recent studies have suggested that the increased frequency of urinary infection in infant boys may be related to the uncircumcised foreskin, under which bacteria may grow. However, these findings must be confirmed by other studies before recommending routine circumcision to decrease the risk of urinary infection.

In the past, some physicians felt that many young girls who seemed susceptible to urinary infections had an abnormally narrow urethra. As a result of this, many young girls were subjected to stretching of the urethra (called urethral dilatation), usually under general anesthesia. We now believe that urethral size in females is not a factor in urinary infection and that there is no reason to stretch the urethra in an attempt to manage urinary tract infections in girls.

Signs and Symptoms of Urinary Tract Infections

The signs and symptoms of urinary infections in children vary with age. Infants usually do not demonstrate the typical symptoms that occur in older children. Instead, they may be irritable, feed and gain weight poorly, or have vomiting or diarrhea. Since infants with these general symptoms will more commonly have other illnesses, the possibility of a urinary infection is often overlooked. As a child reaches toddler age, fever often occurs with urinary infection. The possibility of urinary infection must be considered if an unexplained fever occurs in a toddler who is not yet speaking and is not yet toilet trained. Although urinary infections are readily diagnosed after the age of 3, many infections in younger children may be missed because of lack of specific symptoms.

After toilet training occurs and when a child can speak, it becomes easier to recognize a urinary tract infection. Children may complain of a burning sensation when urinating (*dysuria*) or of pain in the lower stomach area. Other signs may include more frequent or more urgent urination, as well as accidental pants-wetting (*enuresis*). More than half of children with these symptoms, however, do not actually have a urinary infection. These symptoms may also result from other causes of irritation of the urethra, such as bubble baths, poor hygiene, constipation, or tight underclothes. The only reliable way to diagnose a urinary tract infection is by a urine culture.

In addition to the above symptoms, children with infections in the kidney (pyelonephritis) are more likely to have high fever. Older children may also complain of side or back pain. Nausea and vomiting occur more commonly in children with pyelonephritis than in those with a simple bladder infection.

Making the Diagnosis of a Urinary Infection

As we have discussed, the symptoms of a urinary tract infection, especially in the young child, may not be specific. Furthermore, many children with urinary complaints will not have an infection. A screening test for urinary infection that can be performed in a physician's office is a urinalysis, in which the urine is examined chemically and under the microscope. This can be helpful in calling attention to children who might be infected, but urinalysis alone is not sufficient to make a diagnosis. The diagnosis is best made by a urine culture.

A urine culture is performed by placing a small amount of urine into a material that promotes the growth of most bacteria that may be present in the specimen. After 24 hours, the culture is examined for bacteria that might indicate the presence of a urinary tract infection. If necessary, this culture can also be used to find out which antibiotic would be best for treating the infection.

In children who are not yet toilet trained, the urine specimens are usually obtained by applying a small collection bag to the skin around the urethra. If the urine culture from this collection does not have any significant bacteria, the test is usually sufficient. Often, however, the urine is contaminated by skin bacteria. Contamination is directly related to the length of time the collection bag remains applied to the child. If contamination is suspected or the culture is inconclusive, it is advisable to repeat the culture.

Contamination can usually be avoided by collecting a urine specimen with a small plastic tube that is passed through the urethra into the bladder. Another alternative, in infants, is to insert a small needle through the lower abdominal wall directly into the bladder to withdraw a small amount of urine. This may seem excessive for such a simple task as obtaining urine. But the procedure is quite safe, and unfortunately, it is precisely the young children, from whom sterile urine collection is most difficult, who are at greatest risk for complications of urinary infection. Therefore, the extra effort to obtain a good culture is justified and very important for accurate diagnosis.

In older children who are toilet trained, a "midstream" urine specimen can be obtained by urinating into a sterile cup after cleansing the skin around the urethral opening. Even these specimens can easily become contaminated, especially if there is delay between obtaining the specimen and placing it into the culture material. If a delay of more than 30 minutes is expected, the urine specimen should be kept cold in a refrigerator and sent to the laboratory on ice. This will minimize the growth of contaminating bacteria.

Other Types of Evaluation

Over 60% of children who have a first urinary infection will have at least one more. Also, almost half of young children with urinary infections will have an associated abnormality of the urinary tract. Therefore, a careful evaluation of the structure of the urinary tract is warranted in those children who become infected, particularly in all boys, in girls under the age of 7 or 8 years, and in any child with recurring or febrile urinary infections. The goal of this evaluation is to identify abnormalities that could contribute to further infections and to prevent permanent kidney damage.

At our medical center, this evaluation begins with a bladder X ray called a cystogram (see chapter 2). This test may be unpleasant for the child because of the insertion of the catheter into the bladder. But it is important, since about one out of three children with infections of the urine will have a condition known as reflux (or, more accurately, *vesicoureteral reflux*). Reflux refers to the backflow of urine from the bladder into the ureter and up to the kidney (Figure 16). This usually results from a congenital abnormality of the valve where the ureter and bladder meet. This valve normally allows urine to pass freely down into the bladder, while preventing urine from backing up from the bladder into the ureter.

Reflux allows urinary bacteria, which might be causing a simple cystitis, to reach the kidney, where they can cause a more serious pyelonephritis. If reflux is detected, the problem can be treated and further episodes of urinary infection and/or pyelonephritis often can be prevented. This treatment will be discussed later in this chapter.

The cystogram is also important in evaluating boys who have had a urinary infection and who may have been born with partial blockage of the urethra (congenital posterior urethral valves).

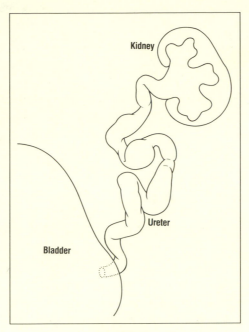

FIGURE 16
Drawing (top) and X ray (bottom) of severe urinary reflux. Free passage of
urine *up* the urinary tract toward the kidney, often associated with urinary
infection, can cause permanent damage to the kidneys (compare with normal X rays of the kidney in chapter 2).

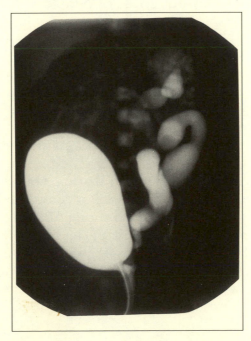

Children with urinary tract infections also should be evaluated with a kidney sonogram or an intravenous pyelogram (see chapter 2). Either of these tests is done to detect blockage of the ureters or other birth defects involving the structure of the urinary system. These types of abnormalities are found in about 5% of children who have had a diagnosed urinary tract infection. The most common site of blockage is where the ureter connects with the kidney (called ureteropelvic junction obstruction). The next most common site of obstruction is where the ureter enters the bladder (called ureterovesical junction obstruction). Generally, obstruction of the kidney will require surgical correction.

If the above tests are abnormal, the child may require further evaluation with a type of renal scan. The scan provides considerable information about the function and drainage of the kidneys. This helps physicians tell the type and severity of the problem that is contributing to the infection.

Potential Consequences of a Urinary Infection

Although simple cystitis may cause temporary discomfort, it rarely causes any serious long-term health problems. However, many children who have had one bladder infection are more likely to have recurrences, suggesting a weakness of the natural defense mechanisms, as mentioned earlier in this chapter.

On the other hand, pyelonephritis in the young child, particularly when associated with reflux, more likely results in permanent scarring of the kidney. The presence of kidney scarring increases the likelihood that the child will develop high blood pressure in adolescence or young adulthood. Depending on the severity of the scarring, high blood pressure may develop in as much as 15% of children with reflux and infection. Also, if the scarring is more extensive and involves both kidneys, progressive kidney failure can occur. More than 10 to 15% of cases of childhood kidney failure are associated with recurring infections of the kidneys.

Treatment of Urinary Infections

Treatment of urinary infections depends upon the type of infection and the presence of possible complicating conditions. Children with simple cystitis can usually be treated with a short course of the safest, least toxic, and least expensive antibiotic to which the bacteria are sensitive. In contrast, urinary infections with fever or other symptoms of pyelonephritis may require hospitalization and intravenous antibiotics, at least for part of the treatment course. Often, children who have not been tested previously will be kept on antibiotics until the X-ray tests are obtained and evaluated.

Some children will have repeated episodes of urinary infection for no obvious reason. Some of these children can be successfully treated with continuous low doses of antibiotic medication for months, or even years, to reduce the frequency of infection. These children are often helped by a regular voiding schedule, emptying the bladder every 3 to 4 hours. The recurrent infections often disappear when the child enters puberty. If no kidney damage was present at the time of initial evaluation and the infections were controlled, these children are not at great risk for serious problems in the future.

For children with reflux, the treatment plan will vary according to the child's age, the number of urinary tract infections, and the X-ray findings. Reflux is measured on a scale of 1 through 5, where grade 1 is the mildest and grade 5 is the most severe. In children with mild to moderate grades of reflux (grades 1 to 3), there is an excellent chance that the reflux will disappear as the child gets older and not be associated with permanent kidney damage. Therefore, many of these children can be managed without surgery.

Conservative treatment of children with mild reflux is possible because it requires both reflux and urinary tract infection to produce kidney damage. A low dose of a safe antibiotic can be given to prevent urinary tract infection for as long as the reflux is present. The medication does not cure the reflux, but it decreases the risk of urinary infection that could lead to kidney scarring. Thousands of children have been treated for long periods of time on this type of program. It has been proved to be safe and effective when the medication is given daily, although approximately 5 to 10% of these children will develop a "breakthrough" infection while on antibiotics. This may require more aggressive treatment.

It is also necessary to obtain periodic bladder X rays to re-evaluate the reflux and to check for the disappearance of the reflux. Once this has happened, the treatment with daily antibiotics can be discontinued.

Reflux can also be surgically corrected. The operation is safe and effective, with a success rate of more than 95% when done by surgeons who perform it often. We usually recommend surgery for children who have the higher degrees of reflux (grades 4 and 5), who have breakthrough infections while on medical treatment, or who continue to have moderate reflux when they approach adolescence. However, factors influencing the decision to operate in individual patients vary and require a careful discussion with the urologist who evaluates your child.

In conclusion, it is important to diagnose and treat urinary tract infections as early and as completely as possible. This is the best way to prevent severe or frequent infections that can damage the urinary tract and the kidneys. If congenital problems lead to urine backing up into the kidneys (reflux), further evaluation and treatment with long-term antibiotics or surgery can prevent kidney scarring.

Chapter 5
Chronic Kidney Failure

As discussed in chapter 1, the kidney performs many different functions, including (1) removing the waste products produced by normal metabolism, (2) regulating the balance of water and minerals in response to the amount a person eats or drinks, (3) reclaiming important substances so that they may be reused by the body, and (4) producing certain hormones that affect such functions as blood pressure, bone structure, and production of red blood cells. Although there are diseases in which only one of these functions is abnormal, the term "kidney failure" is used when all of them, to one degree or another, have malfunctioned.

Acute and Chronic Kidney Failure

When kidney failure starts suddenly, it is called acute renal (kidney) failure. The term "acute" means the kidney injury appears and progresses over a brief period of time, such as days or a week. Chronic kidney failure is often the result of injury that occurs over a longer period of time, such as months to years.

The terms "acute" and "chronic" also relate to the possibility that the kidney failure will go away. Individuals with acute kidney failure may regain normal kidney function once the condition causing injury to the kidney is gone and the kidney has had time to heal. However, individuals with chronic kidney failure usually have kidney malfunction that is permanent and will not get better with time. Although most children with "acute" kidney failure recover fully, some will not or may regain only a part of their kidney function. Such children are then considered to have been left with "chronic" or permanent kidney failure, even though they started with what seemed like acute or temporary kidney failure.

Chronic kidney failure may occur at any time during a person's life. For example, if obstruction to the drainage of urine from the kidney occurs during the development of the fetus in the uterus, the baby may have chronic kidney failure at birth (see chapter 3). In contrast, an otherwise healthy child may develop chronic kidney failure as a result of glomerulonephritis later in life.

Diagnosis of Kidney Failure

The presence of kidney failure is generally diagnosed by the measurement in the child's blood of increased amounts of waste products, which would normally have been eliminated from the body by the kidney. As discussed in chapter 2, blood creatinine and urea are two waste products that are easily measured in all laboratories. Generally, the higher the blood creatinine, the worse the kidney function. Blood urea is a less accurate indicator of kidney function, since its level can be significantly affected by such things as the amount of food eaten, the type of food eaten, and whether the child is dehydrated. By measuring blood creatinine, your child's doctor can estimate the degree of kidney failure with reasonable accuracy. Other blood, urine, and radiological tests are often necessary to diagnose kidney failure and to estimate its degree, but the measurement of blood creatinine is one of the most widely used because of its ready availability.

Although the blood creatinine indicates the presence of renal failure, the degree to which the creatinine is elevated does not indicate whether the kidney disease will get better. Many children with acute kidney failure will have very elevated creatinine levels but may still go on to recover. Rather, the elevation of creatinine and urea (the amount of excess waste products that have accumulated in the blood) is related to the development of symptoms of kidney failure.

Symptoms and Signs of Kidney Failure

Many children with kidney failure will develop "symptoms" (what the child experiences) and "signs" (what others can see in the child) as a result of kidney failure. These signs and symptoms of kidney failure collectively are termed *uremia*. It is possible for kidney failure to be detectable by blood tests but be so mild that the child has no symptoms.

Symptoms of uremia affect many parts of the body. The most obvious effects are on the nervous system and the intestinal tract. Often there are changes in behavior so that a child who was pleasant previously may become irritable, demanding, and difficult to deal with. Thinking processes are generally slowed, and the child may do less well in school and lose interest in activities that formerly were important. Muscular coordination may be impaired as reflected in difficulty with actions that require fine motor skills or in a deterioration in handwriting. The combination of uremia and the anemia that usually accompanies kidney failure may make the child tire more easily, resulting in longer naps or falling asleep in school.

With uremia the child's appetite often becomes poor, and vomiting or diarrhea may occur. Poor feeding and vomiting are particularly common problems in infants with kidney failure. As a result the child or infant may gain weight slowly or may lose weight. Poor nutrition may result in low-quality growth of hair and nails, and in the development of vitamin deficiencies. In addition, skin color may become pale or sallow in appearance, particularly if the child has more severe anemia.

Somewhat less obvious, but equally important, are the effects of chronic kidney failure on the heart and bones. Elevated levels of blood potassium, a common mineral in the normal diet, may lead to dangerous abnormalities in heartbeat. High levels of waste products may cause inflammation of the tissues that surround the heart, leading to fluid collection. If high blood pressure is present, it may put an added strain on the heart, causing it to pump less effectively, which may lead to heart failure.

As discussed in chapter 1, the kidneys are important in the regulation of blood calcium and phosphorus levels, and in the activation of vitamin D. In chronic kidney failure the phosphorus that is normally absorbed from food the child eats is not removed from the body in an efficient manner, and thus the level of phosphorus in the blood rises. This causes the blood calcium level to fall. These abnormalities may lead to such symptoms and signs as nausea and "shakiness." If the calcium level falls too low there is a danger of muscle cramps and spasm or a convulsion. Furthermore, the calcium and phosphorus abnormalities, combined with inefficient activation of vitamin D, often lead to poorly formed bone. Such abnormal bone formation coupled with poor nutrition and other less clearly understood factors may result in poor growth. Bones that bear the child's weight may become less rigid, causing them to bend under their load. These children may complain of joint or bone pain, and they may develop bowlegs or other skeletal deformities. If this persists for a long time, damage may be done to the joints, and growth may be permanently stunted.

There are other, even more subtle effects of chronic kidney failure. The immune system in children with chronic kidney failure functions less well and does not react to infections as promptly or efficiently as in healthy children. In addition, their bodies do not interact with many medications in the same way as the body of a child with normal kidney function. These children may develop side effects from doses of medications that they would ordinarily tolerate if their kidney function were normal.

Factors That Determine if a Child Will Have Symptoms and Signs

Although all children with kidney failure have elevated levels of waste products in their blood, the types and severity of symptoms and signs will vary from child to child. In general, the symptoms and signs will be affected by three factors: the type of kidney disease, its severity, and the length of time it has been present.

As discussed in chapter 3, all kidney diseases that can result in kidney failure can be divided into two general groups: those that predominantly injure the inner part of the kidney, causing more damage to the tubules of the nephrons than to the glomeruli (filters); and those that injure the outer part of the kidney, causing more damage to the glomeruli than to the tubules.

The principal functions associated with the tubules are to reabsorb water, minerals, and other chemicals; to eliminate acid waste from the body; to secrete certain hormones such as erythropoietin; and to activate vitamin D. Infants and children with more damage to tubules than to glomeruli will tend to make large amounts of urine each day and to lose in that urine many of the minerals and other chemicals that normally would have been reclaimed. Although these children seem to urinate a lot, the urine is mostly water and dissolved minerals, with only small amounts of waste products. Because of the mineral and water loss, these children rarely have high blood pressure or swelling. However, they often have more severe anemia and worse bone disease. Conditions that can cause this type of kidney damage include obstruction of urine flow with destruction of the central parts of the kidney and the tubules, as well as various cystic diseases and damage from kidney infections.

The other general group of symptoms results from diseases that cause more damage to the glomeruli than to the tubules. In this case the child usually makes only small amounts of urine each day. These children often have high blood pressure (and its accompanying symptoms), and many will have swelling, particularly around the eyes or in the ankles and feet. Although they also usually have anemia and bone disease, these abnormalities generally do not become severe until later, compared to their progression in children who have more tubular damage. Conditions that most often cause this group of symptoms include inflammation of the glomeruli (glomerulonephritis) and scarring of the glomeruli (*glomerulosclerosis*).

In reality, most chronic kidney failure usually results from some combination of both glomerular and tubular damage. Nonetheless, the symptoms related to more severe damage in one area than the other often are more obvious. This concept explains how two different children may have the same degree of kidney failure, even though one makes only a little urine and the other makes a normal or an excessive amount of urine.

This concept is also important in designing a treatment program. For instance, the infant with primarily tubular damage may need extra fluid and certain minerals in the diet to replace those lost by the abnormal kidney function. However, if extra fluid and minerals are given to a child who has mostly glomerular damage, swelling and hypertension will often develop. The prescription of the amount of fluid and minerals required must be individually determined for each child by the doctor. The wrong treatment program may make the child more ill. Furthermore, the child's needs may change as the disease progresses or the child grows. It often takes repeated laboratory tests and physical examinations to determine the best treatment program. It is important for parents to follow carefully the advice of their child's doctor in these matters.

A second important factor that affects symptoms and signs is the severity of the kidney failure. To better understand this factor let us look at the concept of various degrees of kidney function. Normal people of all ages should have 100% of the kidney function that is normal for that age. Since "normal" kidney function may vary from person to person, it is more practical to think of normal kidney function as being within a range of normal to allow for this variation.

The range of normal kidney function is usually considered to vary from 80 to 120% of the average at any particular age. Kidney function between 50 and 80% of normal is generally considered to represent mild kidney failure, that between 20 and 50% is moderate in severity, and 10 to 20% is severe in degree. Renal function less than 10% of normal usually is insufficient to sustain life for very long. Kidney function that is less than 10% is often referred to as "end-stage renal disease." The term "end-stage" implies a permanent loss of kidney function that is so severe that for the person to continue to live he or she must receive dialysis treatments or a kidney transplant (see chapter 6).

Chronic kidney failure may remain the same in degree (be static) or get worse (be progressive). Kidney failure that gets worse may do so for several reasons. First of all, the condition that is causing the kidney failure may still be present and active. An example is a child who has obstructed kidneys in whom the obstruction has not been corrected. Second, some of the consequences of kidney failure may be inadequately controlled. These consequences may themselves make the kidney failure worse. An example of this is when poor control of high blood pressure may itself make the kidney failure worse. The importance of this concept has become well recognized in recent years.

Also, even if the kidney disease is no longer active and the consequences are well controlled, the child may outgrow what kidney function there is left. In this latter case, the kidney is working as hard as it can, but it cannot keep up with the needs of the body as the child gets bigger. The course of chronic kidney failure, whether it is static or progressive, will vary from child to child. Only a series of physical examinations and laboratory tests can determine each child's pattern.

Finally, the length of time the chronic kidney failure is present influences which child will have symptoms and signs. For example, moderate kidney failure over a number of years may slowly produce severe bone deformities. In contrast, severe kidney failure of only weeks' duration, while associated with abnormalities of calcium and phosphorus, will not cause significant bone disease. In chronic kidney failure the development of bone disease takes time.

Treatment for Kidney Failure

The treatment program for each child must be individualized according to all the factors mentioned above. Obviously, the best treatment program can be decided on only after all of the necessary diagnostic information is available.

There are four general aims of treatment. First, any kidney failure abnormalities that are life-threatening must be treated immediately. Second, circumstances that may cause the kidney injury to get worse should, if possible, be treated so that progression of the disease can be stopped or at least slowed. Third, the child should be helped to feel better, so that he or she can function as normally as possible under the circumstances. Finally, treatment should be started to minimize any damaging effects of the kidney failure on other organs.

The need for immediate correction of life-threatening problems will usually be obvious from the initial examination and laboratory tests. These treatments take priority. In addition, even very early in the child's evaluation, the doctor will try to determine treatments that can slow the progression of kidney failure as much as possible. Some kidney problems may be "fixable," such as blocked urine drainage that can be corrected surgically. Other situations may be "treatable," such as high blood pressure that can be controlled with medications and diet. As already mentioned, treatment of these consequences of chronic kidney failure is important, because if they are left untreated they may speed the rate at which kidney failure gets worse. Information on what "fixable" and "treatable" problems a child has will become evident to the doctor as the diagnostic evaluation of the child progresses.

Treatment of the damaging effects of kidney failure centers on attempting to mimic those functions that, under normal circumstances, the kidneys would have done automatically. Every plan must include provisions for fluid intake, nutritional intake, and medications specific for certain problems. Generally, during treatment the child should be encouraged to maintain as normal a level of activity as possible, including school attendance and physical activity. Your child's doctor will help determine your child's optimal level of activity.

Since the kidney usually regulates the fluid content of the body, we normally think little about the amount of fluid we drink. In the child with kidney failure, the amount of fluid ingested becomes very important, particularly in young infants who cannot complain of thirst or in children whose capacity to get rid of excess fluid is limited. The desired amount of fluid will be decided by your child's doctor depending on your child's needs. As mentioned before, these needs may change over time.

Nutrition is a very important and complicated part of every treatment program for kidney failure. It is particularly important in children, who, unlike adults, must be provided with enough nutrition to promote normal growth. The type of nutrition is also very important, since certain foods are nutritious and cause only minimal stress for the kidney, while others are equally nutritious but cause the kidney to work harder. The first type of foods are said to have a "higher biological value" and are usually better for the child with kidney failure. In some circumstances, foods containing certain minerals or proteins should be avoided, since a child may have a problem handling that particular substance. Foods containing high levels of potassium, for example, often create problems for children with kidney failure.

Individual diets need to be worked out, sometimes by trial and error, to determine the best possible nutritional combination. Such diets need to take into consideration the food preferences of the child as much as possible, since it does no good to design a diet that is fine in theory but that the child refuses to eat. Parents often need to become more "label conscious," paying attention to the contents of commercially prepared food and drink. An additional factor is that some foods the child particularly enjoys may need to be limited or eliminated.

Implementing the prescribed diet can often be difficult and may become a source of struggle between the child and the parents. Specially trained "renal dietitians," particularly those with experience in pediatric nutrition, can be valuable resources for designing and monitoring the effects of kidney-failure diets. A great deal of study is currently under way in determining how certain dietary changes can modify the progression of chronic kidney disease. Ask your child's doctor about these newer developments and how they may apply to your child.

Medications are often used to counteract other aspects of kidney failure. Phosphorus is present in many foods and is difficult to reduce in the diet without also lowering the nutritional content. Certain medications, taken with meals, may be required to reduce the amount of phosphorus that is absorbed from the bowel. If high blood pressure is a problem, medications can also be given to reduce blood pressure to an acceptable level. Supplements such as calcium and a potent form of vitamin D may also be necessary in many children. Other medications will be prescribed depending on the child's individual needs.

It is the doctor's responsibility to prescribe these medications and to monitor both the good and possible bad effects by regular examinations, blood tests, and X rays. Medication doses must often be adjusted as the degree of kidney failure changes or the child grows. Parents need to work as a team with the doctor under these circumstances. Administration of the medications to infants may be difficult, and older children may resist taking them. Parents should avoid starting any medication, even seemingly harmless nonprescription (over-the-counter) medicines, without consulting their child's doctor. Some of these medicines may have a bad effect on the child or worsen kidney function. In addition, certain medicines need to be given in reduced dosage or at longer-than-normal intervals when kidney function is abnormal. Your doctor will take these factors into consideration when prescribing or recommending other medications. A more detailed discussion of many of these medication issues can be found in chapter 9.

Helping the child with kidney failure to feel better is the goal of the fluid, diet, and medicine plan, although following the plan may be a challenge for the parents. Having a positive attitude toward the future and being sensitive to the child's concerns are important factors.

It has been our experience that children generally do best if they are well informed and are a central part of the treatment planning process. As much as possible, pediatric patients should be present during conferences with their doctors so that they understand that they are being told the truth about their situation. It is natural for parents to want to protect their child from worry as much as possible. However, withholding the truth from a child who is old enough to understand usually leads to more anxiety, not less. Such "shielded" children often imagine they are sicker and their future is more dismal than their parents and the doctors have told them. As a result, they may become more fearful in general and mistrustful of their parents and other caretakers. This often leads to resistance to treatment and an uncooperative attitude in general.

Many children and their families will need help in coping with these chronic problems. Such help from social workers, psychologists, and psychiatrists is usually readily available in a setting that is attuned to comprehensive pediatric care. Parents should be sensitive to the value of these resources and make use of them whenever necessary, so that family functioning is disrupted as little as possible. This also allows problems in other family members to be identified and resolved earlier, before they become harder to treat.

In many cases successful treatment can prevent or delay further deterioration of kidney function. When this is not possible, the majority of children who develop end-stage renal disease can be helped by dialysis treatments and *transplantation*. These topics are discussed in chapter 6.

Chapter 6

When the Kidneys Fail: Dialysis and Transplantation

Not too many years ago, permanent kidney failure inevitably led to death. Today, some form of dialysis or transplantation can be offered to virtually every child with kidney failure. However, there is still a great need for further progress in these fields. These are not simple treatments, and they require a great deal of time and expense, as well as patience on the part of the family.

Despite this, we have seen many children rise above their medical problems. With expert treatment, family support, perseverance, and a little good fortune, children with kidney failure can grow into active and productive young adults. We'd like to introduce you to Jason and Jennifer, two children who are making the most of their chances for a better life.

Jason is 13 years old. Although he had a congenital abnormality of the kidneys since birth, his kidney disease remained undetected until he was 9. Over the past four years his kidney function tests have slowly worsened. We talked frequently with Jason and his parents about what treatments would be available when his kidneys failed. But Jason felt pretty good, despite his kidney disease. It was very difficult for him when the time finally came to sit down with his family and his doctors to make specific plans about dialysis and transplantation. Although he probably heard what we said all along about the future, it's easy to tell yourself that it won't really happen. Protecting ourselves from bad feelings is just part of being human.

When the time did come, however, Jason and his family were able to consider their treatment options. With the help of doctors, nurses, and many other health professionals, as well as other patients, they were able to make the decisions necessary to go on with life, and to make the most of it.

As kidney function worsens, there comes a time when some form of kidney replacement therapy must be considered—dialysis or kidney transplantation. As discussed in the preceding chapter, when that time occurs is extremely variable from one individual to another. Most nephrologists use two general rules to guide the decision to begin one of these treatments:

1. when the potentially harmful body disturbances caused by the kidney failure are no longer controlled in a satisfactory manner by the use of medication and diet, or
2. when the symptoms of kidney failure are dangerous or seriously interfere with normal daily activities.

Jennifer and her family have been coming to us for many years, and she has received medical treatment, dialysis, and finally transplantation for her kidney failure. On looking back to the early days of her medical care, Jennifer's mother wrote:

"I don't think I really believed Dr. Bock when he told me the extent of Jennifer's renal disease. She didn't look that sick. It was difficult to comprehend that she would someday need dialysis and a transplant. I kept thinking she would get better, or at least not get any worse. Thank God that was all in the future, almost two years; it gave us time to prepare ourselves and realize the extent of her illness."

Often, it is difficult for people close to the patient to see the changes that occur with progressive kidney failure. Jennifer's mom was no exception:

"The next two years Jennifer slowly deteriorated. It was difficult for me to detect at times because it was so slow and so many of the signs could be attributed to teenage behavior. But I

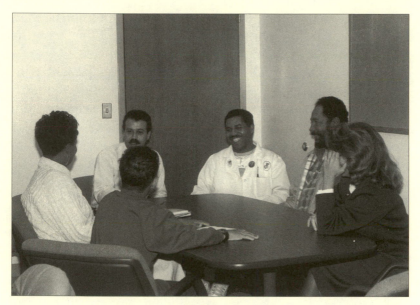

FIGURE 17
The meeting between members of the health care team and the family is intended to be an opportunity for the parents and patient to participate in important decisions relating to selection of kidney failure treatment options. Meeting in this manner often aids effective two-way communication between doctors and patients.

couldn't deny some of them. Her gait became much worse, she slept most of the time, she did things haphazardly if at all, and she was so irritable. The medication list got longer and longer, and she developed hypertension. The time for dialysis had arrived.''

When a patient faces the need to select a type of kidney failure treatment, the physician, nurse, and social worker generally meet with the patient (if he or she is old enough) and the parents. At this meeting, the types of available treatments are discussed and considered. It is not the intent of this chapter to describe, in detail, all aspects of the treatments available for kidney failure. As you can see in the Resources section of this book, there are many places from which information on this subject can be obtained. Rather, we will attempt to present an overview of the various types of treatments and the strengths and weaknesses of each.

Our goal is to provide the parent and older patient with information that will enable them to work confidently with the physicians, nurses, and social workers in selecting the treatment that best fits the needs and desires of the patient and family. It is often useful to begin these discussions when kidney function is worsening but before the patient develops worsening symptoms. This will allow time for careful treatment planning. Keep in mind that not all treatment facilities can always offer all forms of treatments, particularly for small children. If your physician cannot provide a type of treatment in which you have interest, be sure to ask who you can talk to about such treatments.

Kidney Dialysis

The term "dialysis" refers to one of several treatment techniques, each of which attempts to replace the functions formerly provided by the person's kidneys. These treatments restore the fluid and mineral balance of the body, while removing unnecessary and potentially harmful substances. The use of dialysis not only preserves life in patients whose kidneys have failed, it also often provides an overall improvement in the person's activity and well-being when compared to that person's condition before beginning dialysis.

All current forms of dialysis involve passing water and other substances through a membrane. The membrane is a thin layer of tissue, either natural or artificial, that allows water and dissolved substances to pass through from one side to the other. The principle of how a membrane works is depicted in Figure 18. The types of materials passing into or out of the body, and the efficiency with which this happens can be altered by changing the pressure or the composition of the fluids, either on one or on both sides of the membrane.

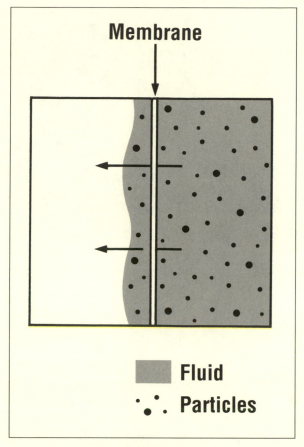

FIGURE 18

The membranes used in peritoneal dialysis (a natural membrane) or hemodialysis (an artificial membrane) share certain common features. As shown in this illustration, water, normal body chemicals, and waste products can pass from one side of the membrane to the other. By controlling the composition of the solutions on the "outside" of the membrane, the types and rates of removal of substances "inside" can, to a great extent, be controlled. This is the fundamental principle of dialysis.

Types of Dialysis

Dialysis may be accomplished using the natural membrane lining the peritoneal (abdominal) cavity, in a process

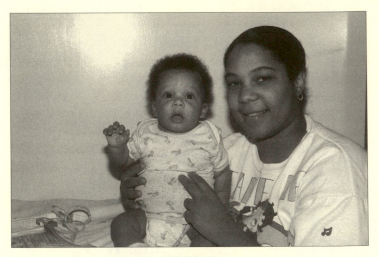

FIGURE 19
Many parents have learned to perform peritoneal dialysis at home
for their infants and children.

called *peritoneal dialysis*. Or, it may be done by passing
the person's blood through an artificial kidney machine that
contains one of several types of manufactured membranes.
This latter process is called *hemodialysis* ("hemo" means
blood).

Peritoneal dialysis has become a widely used form of dialysis treatment. When used to treat chronic renal failure, the
treatments are usually done at home. For the infant and
young child, the dialysis is most often done by a parent or
other adult. Many older children and adolescents can do
their own treatments.

Some parents are concerned that they will not be able to
learn and perform peritoneal dialysis. Although it is natural
to worry about such responsibilities, it is important to realize
that hundreds of parents have had the same insecurities, but
they have ultimately done very well. The people who developed peritoneal dialysis systems made them fairly easy to
use. Parents and patients need only to follow step-by-step
directions carefully, with no shortcuts. These techniques are

taught by skilled hospital personnel who are good at teaching dialysis to all types of people.

If a patient chooses peritoneal dialysis, doctors must surgically insert a clear plastic tube (peritoneal catheter) into the abdomen as is shown in Figure 20. To perform peritoneal dialysis, a solution of sterile water that contains several minerals and other materials is passed through the catheter into the peritoneal cavity. Excessive amounts of substances contained in the blood then can flow through the peritoneal membrane into the dialysis solution. At the same time, other substances the body is lacking can be replenished by passing from the dialysis solution into the blood. Excessive water can be removed from the blood as well, in a process called *ultrafiltration*. After a suitable period of time, the fluid is drained and replaced by fresh solution. This is called a dialysis *exchange*, or *pass.*

Although these are the basic principles used in peritoneal dialysis, there are different ways of actually performing the procedure. As with many things in medicine, these treatments have been given complicated names that describe fairly simple ideas. The two most common types of peritoneal dialysis currently in use are continuous ambulatory peritoneal dialysis (*CAPD*) and continuous cyclic peritoneal dialysis (*CCPD*).

In CAPD, the dialysis solution exchanges are done under sterile conditions throughout the day and night. Generally, four exchanges are done per day—morning, noon, evening, and bedtime. In between these times, the fluid stays in the peritoneal cavity. The dialysis solution is supplied in plastic bags, and the exchanges can be done in any clean area (for example, in the bathroom at home or in the nurse's office at school). When not in use, the bags are either rolled up and placed in an inconspicuous place (like in a pants pocket or under a belt) or they are disconnected.

In CCPD, the exchanges are done by an automatic machine, usually throughout the night. Typically, at bedtime a supply of solution is placed on the machine. While the person is sleeping, the machine regulates the inflow and outflow of the solution, achieving a similar amount of dialysis as

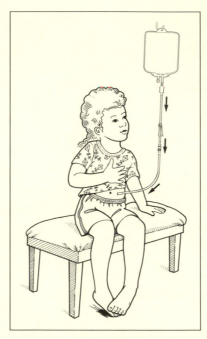

FIGURE 20
Today, there are many variations of the peritoneal dialysis procedure. In one type, fresh sterile fluid is "exchanged" for spent fluid several times a day by removal and replacement through a thin plastic tube.

occurs with CAPD. As with CAPD, the performance of CCPD is done by the patient, family member, or caretaker after suitable training by hospital personnel.

Like CCPD, hemodialysis is also performed using a machine. Some hospitals have programs in which children may receive hemodialysis at home, but most young patients receive their treatments at a medical facility. Although there are several brands of hemodialysis machines, they all basically do the same thing. During a hemodialysis treatment, blood passes out of the body through tubing that is connected to the artificial kidney (Figure 21). These treatments are usually given two to three times per week for two to four hours per treatment. Artificial kidneys also may look different, but they perform similar functions. Blood flows on one

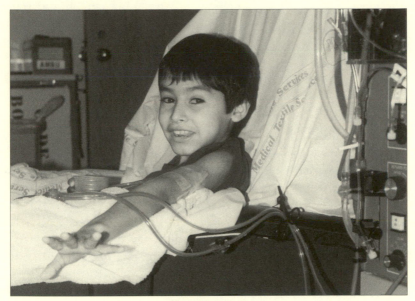

FIGURE 21

During hemodialysis, the blood flows out of the body (the left arm, in this case) via a tube, through the artificial kidney, and back into the body in a continuous circuit.

side of the membrane and dialysis solution on the other. In the same way described for peritoneal dialysis, body fluids and dissolved materials undergo changes as they pass across the membrane. Waste products are removed from the blood and are carried away by the dialysis solution.

In order to provide efficient treatment, the blood must flow rapidly through the artificial kidney. In fact, during the average hemodialysis treatment, the total volume of blood in the body must circulate through the artificial kidney two to three times per hour. To do this accurately and safely, the dialysis machine contains a pump to move the blood at a constant rate, as well as safety devices that monitor the system.

As you can imagine, simply placing two needles in separate veins would not allow the blood to be withdrawn and returned fast enough. This is why special forms of access to the blood vessels (*vascular access*) are needed for hemodialysis. There are many types of vascular access. Most commonly, a surgical connection is made between an artery and a vein to create a system in which blood flow is rapid. Needles can be placed into this surgical connection and blood circulated through them. When the blood vessels are directly connected, most commonly in the forearm, this is called a *fistula*.

Small children have blood vessels that are usually too small for a fistula connection. In this case, a piece of artificial blood vessel can be inserted between the artery and vein, usually in the upper arm or leg. This is called a *graft*. In addition, several types of catheters can be placed through the skin into a large blood vessel. Many are divided down the middle in the inside so that dialysis can be performed through them without the need to insert a needle with each treatment. The specific pros and cons of different types of vascular access should be discussed with your physicians in order to decide which is best for your child.

What Dialysis Can and Can't Do

There are two very important things to realize about dialysis. First, it is a substitute for failed kidney function—it will not make the kidneys better when the problem is chronic renal failure. Second, while many patients find that they begin to feel better after a settling-in period on dialysis, it is unrealistic to expect to feel perfectly healthy from the treatments. In fact, some people will experience cramps, nausea, or vomiting during the hemodialysis treatment.

Although all forms of dialysis can maintain the balance of minerals, water, and waste products in the body well enough to prevent serious complications, dialysis is a poor substitute for our own kidneys. Even at its best, dialysis provides only about 10% of the overall normal filtering capacity of human kidneys. But that seems to be a sufficient amount of artificial function to enable many youngsters and adults to live active, productive lives.

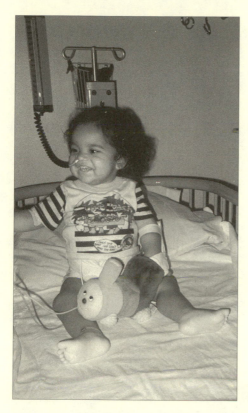

Austin Lee is all smiles when his
mom arrives at the hospital after work.

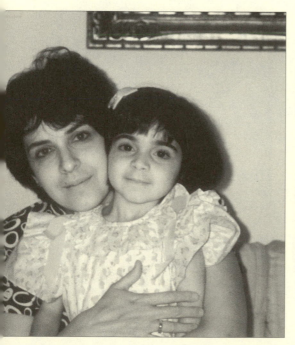

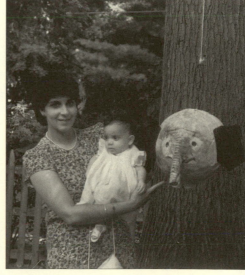

Eugenia has had kidney failure since
infancy. Her mother took advantage
of every opportunity for "quality time"
together (right). Even though Eugenia
has become a young lady, she obviously
still enjoys time with her mom (left).

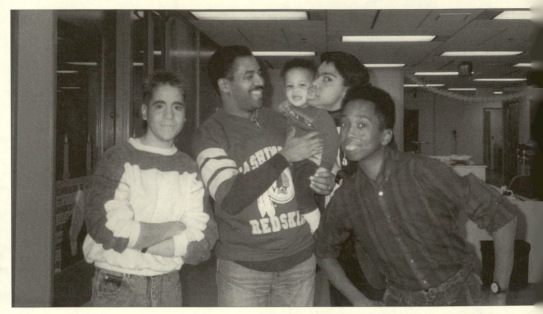

Dialysis nurses like Gerry Todd are often seen as big "brothers" and "sisters" by many of the dialysis patients.

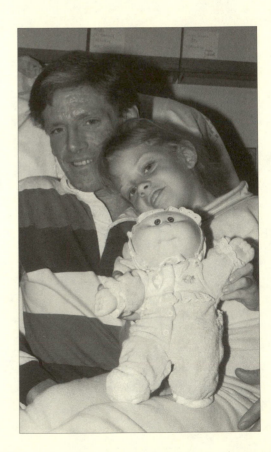

Kim Fisher is happy to have her dad with her during her outpatient examinations.

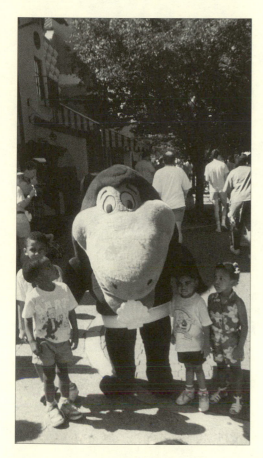

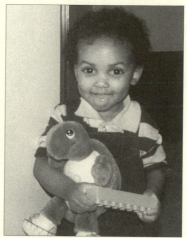

Michael shows off a new friend (above), which he "won" during a nephrology patient trip to a local amusement park (left).

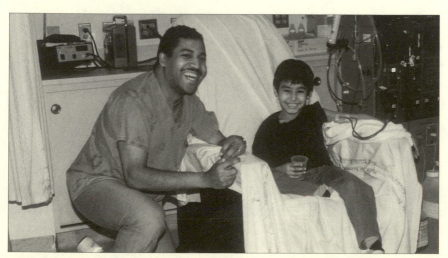

Willie Lopez can always be counted on to bring a big smile to the dialysis unit.

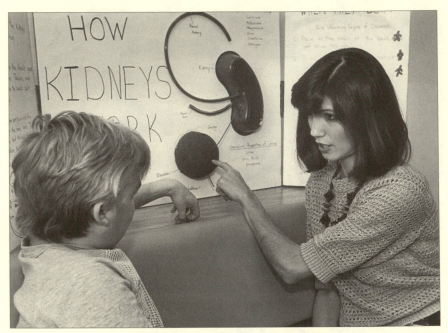

Social worker Camille Bock points out some kidney "basics" to a patient considering transplantation.

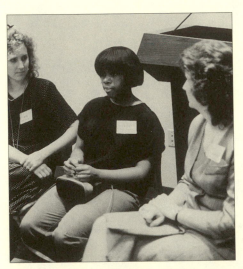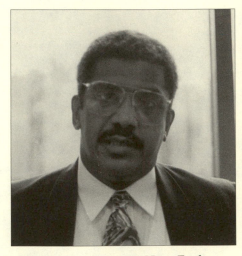

Education of the public about kidney disease in childhood is important. Here, Fred Blanchard (right) explains to a group of Kidney Foundation volunteers what it was like to donate a kidney to his daughter, Kim. Social worker Kim O'Connor and dialysis nurse Kathleen Riley look on as patient Tanita Simmons (left-center) relates to the group what it is like to be on dialysis while continuing to attend school.

You may recall from chapter 1 that healthy kidneys also perform other important functions, including the regulation of blood pressure, calcium balance, and production of red blood cells. These functions are also imperfectly provided by dialysis. Therefore, while on dialysis, most patients must continue to receive medications and dietary guidance similar to those discussed in the previous chapter.

Which Type of Dialysis Is Best?

The answer to this question is subject to many opinions. The patient and the family must weigh several factors in determining their preference. One important consideration is in which type of dialysis your physician has the greatest expertise. Other considerations include the age and motivation of the patient, type of underlying disease, family characteristics, and future treatment goals. In our experience, every case is different. Many factors must be considered to determine what we feel would be the best recommendation for a specific family.

However, there are some important characteristics of the different types of dialysis. The first consideration is who is responsible for providing the treatments. The medical staff is responsible for providing hemodialysis treatments for most children. As we discussed, peritoneal dialysis is usually performed by the patient or family member at home. Although there usually are fewer routine visits to the hospital compared to hemodialysis, actual hospitalization time may be greater for peritoneal dialysis patients. This is because the success of the procedure depends upon performing the dialysis the proper way, every day. A sloppy or casual attitude, or poor home supervision of young patients can result in inadequate treatments. Inattention can also result in frequent, potentially serious infections in the tissue surrounding the peritoneal catheter (*tunnel infection*) or within the abdomen (*peritonitis*).

A second consideration is the time commitment required by the different types of dialysis. If peritoneal dialysis is performed or supervised by a parent, it requires a significant time commitment. This can create problems for the working parent, or for one who has other extensive household responsibilities. By contrast, hemodialysis requires a different type of major time commitment. For the school-age child undergoing treatment at a medical facility, there can be a significant loss of education time, which can lead to poor school performance, limited peer contact, and loss of self-esteem. For the parent of a young child, or for a family that lives far from the hospital, commuting time can be considerable.

A third consideration is the procedure itself. Many pediatric nephrologists believe that the sudden adjustment of body fluids and chemistry over several hours, as is done with hemodialysis, is just not as gentle a procedure as doing the same thing over a longer period of time, as with peritoneal dialysis. As a result, patients may feel "washed out" immediately following a hemodialysis treatment. It is important to realize that treatments such as hemodialysis depend on a successful partnership between the treatment team, who must do their utmost with each procedure, and the patient, who has the responsibility of following diet and medication directions. It is difficult to ignore the temptation of fast-food french fries or a pizza at a friend's house. In general, peritoneal dialysis patients require fewer medications and diet restrictions than do hemodialysis patients. Many patients also object to the needle sticks of each hemodialysis treatment. On the other hand, peritoneal dialysis patients often have trouble adjusting to having a tube coming out of their belly. A comparison of the common forms of dialysis can be seen in Table 2.

In conclusion, there is no single answer to the question, "Which form of dialysis is best?" The advantages and disadvantages must be discussed with your physician and weighed for each individual family. We feel a very important step in the decision-making process is to have the patient meet others undergoing the different types of treatments.

Table 2. Comparison of types of dialysis

Considerations	In-center hemodialysis	CCPD	CAPD
Surgery	Minor surgery needed to make an access, usually in the arm.	Minor surgery needed to place a catheter (small tube) near your navel.	Minor surgery needed to place a catheter (small tube) near your navel.
Independence	Your treatment is given by trained professional staff in a dialysis unit.	You are trained to do the treatment yourself or with a family member.	You are trained to do the treatment yourself or with a family member.
Flexibility	You must travel to a unit for treatment.	The treatment is done in your home, using your own machine.	Treatment can be done in many places. You don't have to stay at home or go to a dialysis unit.
	You must follow the unit's treatment schedule.	Treatment can be done while you are sleeping.	You wear a bag and carry extra bags of dialysate for exchanges.
Equipment	You must be connected to a machine.	You must be connected to a machine.	No machine.
	Needles are used.	No needles are used. The catheter stays in place between treatments.	No needles. The catheter stays in place between treatments.
Diet	Usually more diet restrictions than with peritoneal dialysis.	Fewer diet restrictions than with hemodialysis.	Fewer diet restrictions than with hemodialysis.
Other considerations	Higher risk of hepatitis.	Less risk of hepatitis, but you are subject to peritonitis (an inflammation of the abdominal lining).	Less risk of hepatitis, but you are subject to peritonitis (an inflammation of the abdominal lining).
Appearance changes	The access in your arm is hardly noticeable.	A small tube protrudes from your abdomen, but it is under your clothing.	A small tube protrudes from your abdomen, but it is under your clothing. The fluid may increase the size of your abdomen.
Effectiveness	Each treatment takes 3 to 5 hours. Patients usually need 3 treatments every week. You may have symptoms between treatments as wastes build up in your body.	A treatment takes 10-12 hours and is usually done every night while you sleep. This controls the buildup of wastes better.	Treatment is continuous. Most effective dialysis to control buildup of wastes.

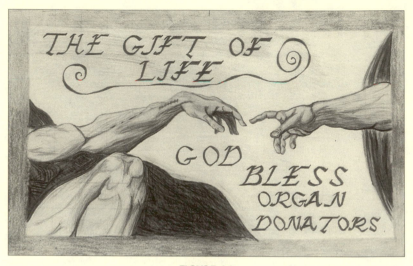

FIGURE 22
An entry in the National Gift of Life Poster and Essay Contest.

This often leads to better understanding and diminished fear of various aspects of the treatments.

Kidney Transplantation

Transplantation means the transfer of body tissue from one place to another. In the case of the kidney, transplantation refers to the removal of a kidney from one person and its surgical placement into another. Although the idea of transferring parts of the body from one person to another has been around for hundreds of years, it is only recently that advances in medical science have allowed this to become a reality.

What makes transplantation so complicated is our old friend, the immune system (see chapter 3). The immune system protects the body from invading bacteria and viruses mainly by recognizing what is "self" and what is not—and by attacking the "not." With the exception of identical twins, we are all different. Therefore, when a kidney is transplanted from one individual to another, the immune system senses that this new organ is "different" and may resist its presence in much the same way that it resists the presence of infecting organisms. This reaction to the transplanted kidney, commonly referred to as *rejection*, is the major obstacle to successful transplantation today.

How Is Transplantation Done?

For an individual who has decided to be a candidate for kidney transplantation, there are three basic parts of the process: (1) finding a suitable kidney for the individual, (2) performing the surgical procedure, and (3) lifelong medical treatment to prevent loss of the kidney through rejection. We will discuss each of these briefly.

Transplanted kidneys come from two sources: Organs donated for transplantation from someone who has died and organs taken from healthy individuals (usually blood relatives). By far, most transplanted kidneys in general, and about one-half for children come from donors whose organs are still healthy even though the persons have been declared dead because the brain has stopped functioning (brain death).

When the decision is made to seek a kidney from a brain-dead donor, the patient is placed on a waiting list. This is a system whereby people who are awaiting kidneys have information placed into a computer list, which then allows them to be matched with suitable kidneys that become available. The waiting time varies, and it depends upon many factors, including certain laboratory tests, the urgency of the need for transplantation, and the characteristics of the kidneys that become available. Today, it is fair to say that the greatest limiting factor in obtaining a kidney for any given individual is that there are many more people waiting than there are kidneys. It is an unfortunate fact that a significant proportion of the families of people who have died do not

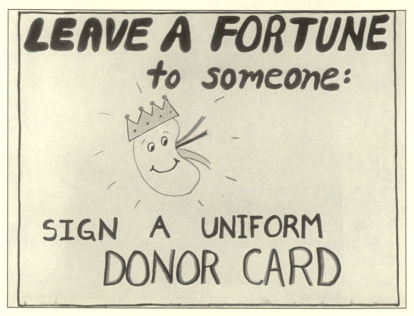

FIGURE 23
An entry in the National Gift of Life Poster and Essay Contest.

give permission to donate the deceased relative's organs for transplantation.

Partly because of this lack of donor kidneys, and also for medical and psychological reasons, living donors continue to contribute a significant portion of the kidneys transplanted to infants and young children. Transplanted kidneys from living donors, on the average, outlast those from cadaver donors. Living donors, most often parents, undergo a detailed medical evaluation to ensure they are in excellent health and are likely to remain so. If this is the case, and if the individual is willing to go through the surgical procedure necessary to donate one of his or her two kidneys, many physicians will go ahead with the transplant.

There is some debate among health care workers as to

whether it is proper to allow a healthy person to assume the risks involved in kidney donation. There is concern about the risk of surgery, as well as the long-term risk of having only one kidney. There is no single right answer to this issue. However, many pediatric centers and parents have viewed living donor transplantation as an important and preferred treatment approach. Based upon currently available information, it seems quite clear that the risks are small enough to justify using kidneys from living donors.

Regardless of who the kidney donor is, there are certain requirements that must be met before considering transplantation. The first requirement is compatibility. Blood group (types A, B, AB, and O) must be compatible between the donor and the recipient (the person receiving the kidney) in the same manner as for blood transfusion (which is actually another form of transplantation!). In addition, the recipient must have serum (the water part of blood that carries chemical products of the immune system) that does not react against tissue from the donor. This test, called the crossmatch, is done just before the actual transplant. If the recipient "reacts" to donor tissue (usually some form of white blood cell) in this test, it means he or she has a high likelihood of immediately rejecting that kidney.

Surgery for the Transplant

In some medical institutions, the surgeon performing the transplant will assume responsibility for later medical care, whereas in others the nephrologist resumes the role of responsible physician after surgery. Most often, the care is jointly assumed by both. If the patient is on a waiting list for a kidney and one becomes available from a donor who has died, the whole process, from evaluation of potential recipients to performance of the actual transplant surgery, is done in as short a period of time as possible. Ideally this is within 24 hours, although, from a practical standpoint, the time period may extend to 48 hours or more. If the patient is receiving a kidney from a living donor, however, the surgery can be scheduled for everyone's convenience.

When the transplant surgery is performed, the kidney is generally placed in the iliac fossa, an area below the abdomen that is partially protected by the pelvic bones (Figure 24). This is often a surprise to many people, who assume that the new kidney would be placed in the same area as one of the failed ones. There are many reasons the procedure is done this way, including the fact that putting the transplant in the area of an old kidney is technically more difficult, requires much more extensive surgery, and would first require the removal of the diseased kidney. Also, placing the transplant in the iliac fossa makes it more accessible to physical examination and biopsy in the case of suspected rejection. The transplant artery and vein are connected to one of several large blood vessels in this area, and the ureter is surgically connected to the bladder.

Most often, the patient's own poorly functioning diseased kidneys do not have to be removed. The decision of whether the diseased kidneys are to be removed or whether other surgery is necessary prior to the transplant will be discussed with you by your transplant physician or surgeon.

Following the transplant surgery, the kidney may not work immediately. The kidney may require a period of healing after being removed from another individual and being in storage. Generally, the longer the time from when the kidney is removed from the donor to when it is transplanted into the recipient, the greater the likelihood of an initial period of no function. Most kidneys that do not initially function following a satisfactory procedure will eventually begin to work.

Medical Treatment of the Transplant

Regardless of how well the transplant works immediately following surgery, it is necessary for virtually all recipients to continue taking antirejection medications for the rest of their

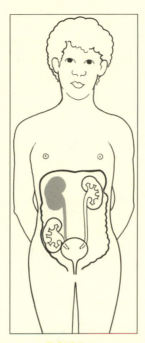

FIGURE 24

Location of the transplanted kidney in most individuals. For reference, the
normal positions of the kidneys are shown. Whether or not the patient's
own kidneys are removed prior to transplantation depends upon a number
of factors, which can be discussed with your nephrologist and transplant surgeon.

lives. These medications, in one way or another, reduce the
sensitivity of the immune system, thereby decreasing the
risk of rejection. This process of controlling the immune system, however, also results in an increased risk for serious
infection—the major complication of transplantation. A description of the more common medications used in transplantation can be found in chapter 9.

Over the past 20 years, numerous medical approaches to
improving the outcome of transplantation have been developed. This has resulted in a gradually and continually improving success rate. Among transplant physicians, there is
great optimism that the remaining problems of transplanta-

tion eventually can be solved. Since each year brings new developments in the field, it is not very useful to describe the present state of the art, since it is likely that this will soon become outdated. It is fair to say, however, that the biggest advances have been in the areas of better systems for the preservation and rapid distribution of donor kidneys, and in less toxic, more effective medications to control rejection. In addition, several approaches to preparing recipients for kidneys from living and nonliving donors have improved the results.

The biggest question for parents considering transplantation for their child is the "chance" of success. Success is often described in terms of "kidney survival." In other words, what percent of the kidneys transplanted are still working at some later time? In most circumstances, it is reasonable to expect that more than 80% of kidneys transplanted from nonliving donors, and more than 90% of those from living donors, will still be working after one year. In general, the longer the period of time after the transplant that the kidney has continued to work, the greater the likelihood of continuing to have a functioning kidney. Nonetheless, we tell most families that it is not realistic to expect any transplant to work indefinitely in this day and age. This is because, although many people have enjoyed functioning transplants for many years, most patients cannot completely avoid rejection and other types of injury to the kidney indefinitely.

What Happens if Rejection Occurs?

As we discussed earlier, rejection describes the process that occurs when the immune system attempts to attack the organ, which it recognizes as not belonging in the body. Although rejection occurs frequently, an episode of rejection, fortunately, does not necessarily mean the inevitable loss of the kidney. Once rejection is recognized, changes in your child's treatment program will occur. This typically involves either using higher doses of the usual medicines or adding new medications. Many of these changes cannot be used for long periods of time, either because they will become ineffective or because they will cause serious complications. However, over a short period, these changes in medical treatment often reverse the rejection process.

It is therefore important to recognize rejection as early as possible, so the medical team can begin treatment promptly to minimize damage to the kidney. The signs and symptoms of rejection may include unexplained fever, swelling or tenderness in the area of the transplant, reduced urine production, or worsening hypertension. Rejection might occur more gradually in some patients, however, and early symptoms may be more subtle, or even absent. Often, the earliest sign is the finding of a worsening blood test during a routine transplant clinic checkup. This underscores the importance of regular checkups by the transplant physician—something that is easy to forget when the patient is feeling well.

If rejection or some other complication of transplantation occurs and results in loss of kidney function, most children will return to dialysis. At that point, the patient, family, and physician must decide whether to continue dialysis or make another attempt at transplantation.

Dialysis or Transplantation?

Although both dialysis and transplantation are considered suitable forms of treatment for adults with chronic renal failure, the prevailing attitude among pediatric nephrologists is that in infants and children, transplantation is the preferable long-term choice. This is not to say that children cannot function reasonably well while undergoing dialysis treatments. However, a considerable amount of information has shown better physical and intellectual development as well as psychological and social maturation in children who have ultimately undergone transplantation compared to those receiving long-term dialysis. These facts must be weighed against the medical condition unique to a given child, the fears of

TO MY DONOR

I don't know if you were male or female,
I don't know if you were young or old.
I do know you must have been
a kind, generous, and giving person.
Someone who cared about others.
To me, you are a hero.

FIGURE 25
An entry in the National Gift of Life Poster and Essay
Contest.

transplant failure, and the sometimes considerable risks of
the transplant surgery and subsequent treatment.

Over the past several years, we have had the opportunity
to spend a great deal of time with young dialysis and transplant patients from around the country during our annual
National Gift of Life Poster and Essay Contest (cosponsored
with the National Kidney Foundation). These creative young
people have given us a great deal of insight through their art
and essays. We have shared several of many excellent examples of their work throughout this chapter.

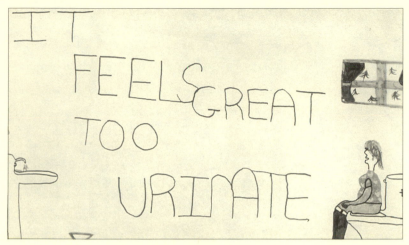

FIGURE 26
An entry in the National Gift of Life Poster and Essay Contest.

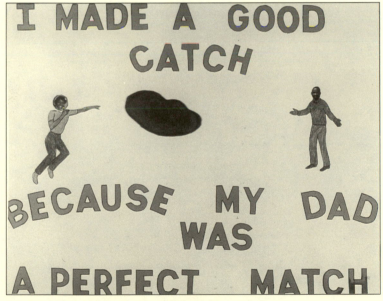

FIGURE 27
An entry in the National Gift of Life Poster and Essay Contest.

Chapter 7
Some Useful
Dietary
Guidelines

This chapter provides a short outline of common types of dietary modifications that may be prescribed for people with kidney disorders. It was written with the assistance of Ann Abbott, R.D.

This information is intended only as an introduction to many of the diet-related terms you might hear from your physician or dietitian. Keep in mind that the type of diet prescribed often is individualized for each patient. The specifics will depend on the type of kidney disorder and the degree of kidney dysfunction. The diet of the patient in the earlier stages of kidney disease is frequently very different from the one of the patient who, for example, is undergoing dialysis treatments.

To best understand your diet and to receive detailed written information, you should consult with a registered dietitian (R.D.). This member of the health care team will discuss your needs with your physician. Together they will determine the best dietary prescription. The dietitian will also review your regular diet and help you make appropriate changes.

Management of the diet is one of the more important, yet difficult responsibilities facing kidney patients and their families. Some of the important terms the dietitian will discuss are fluid, sodium, potassium, protein, and phosphorus. We will discuss the importance of each of these and provide lists of foods that may be important in controlling the

balance of these substances when the kidneys do not function normally. These lists are by no means complete, and
they can be supplemented by information from your physician and dietitian.

Fluid

The kidneys normally regulate the amount of fluid we drink
that remains in our bodies. When the kidneys no longer
function properly, fluid (urine) excretion may be excessive or
inadequate. Either situation may occur, depending on the
type of kidney disorder. Excessive loss of fluid usually is a
problem only for infants, since older children can ask for
something to drink if they are losing too much water. More
commonly, people with kidney disorders have a tendency to
retain too much fluid. The effects of fluid retention on blood
pressure and heart function are discussed in chapter 1.

The physician or dietitian often will prescribe a "fluid restriction" based upon a daily estimate of the amount of fluid
an individual can tolerate with minimal ill effects. Foods that
are liquid at room temperature or that become liquid once ingested are counted as fluids. Milk, soda, water, ice, juice, ice
cream, soup, and flavored gelatins all are examples of fluids.
You must also consider foods that contain a large amount of
fluid. Examples of such foods are watermelon, canned fruits
with syrup, puddings, and yogurt.

Sodium

Excessive sodium ingestion can in itself worsen fluid balance
and blood pressure. In addition, eating foods with a high sodium content also causes thirst, which makes fluid restriction much more difficult. Thirst is a very powerful feeling
and difficult to ignore.

Sodium is a mineral. It is a natural part of many foods,

but its major source is common salt (sodium chloride). Each teaspoon of salt contains approximately 2,000 milli-grams (mg) of sodium. The amount of natural sodium varies from one food to another. For example, milk has a much higher natural sodium content than fruit. Some foods, such as many canned soups, bacon, and pickles, have a great deal of so-dium added either for flavor or as a preservative. Other foods, such as gravies, sauces, casseroles, pot pies, many fast foods, and frozen dinners often contain large amounts of sodium, which may not be obvious when eaten. It is impor-tant to realize that some foods contain considerable sodium even though they do not taste salty.

The average American has acquired a "taste" for high-so-dium foods. This is not something we are born with; infants do not show a preference for salty taste. Just as many of us have "learned" to prefer salty foods, we are capable of "unlearning" that behavior. When starting out, a sodium-limited diet can be difficult to follow since people often miss the "salty" taste of food. However, after an initial adjustment period of four to eight weeks, most people learn to appreciate the natural flavor of foods. Foods with excess sodium begin to taste too salty! To make the transition to a low-salt diet easier, learn to use lemon juice, onion, garlic, herbs, and spices to flavor food. Finally, as a result of public demand, the number of low-sodium products available at reasonable prices has increased in the past few years. Remember, to make an effective diet change such as this, the whole family must participate. Using less salt will generally be a healthy dietary change for everyone. Do not use a salt sub-stitute unless it has been discussed with your physician or dietitian because these products may contain large amounts of potassium.

Examples of foods particularly high in sodium are listed in Table 3.

Potassium

Potassium (often referred to as "K") is a mineral that is es-

Table 3. Foods generally high in sodium

Meat, fish, and cheese

canned, salted, or smoked meats and fish	corned beef
luncheon meats	hot dogs
bacon	sausage
Chinese food	ham
kosher meats	canadian bacon
fast foods	processed cheeses
fatback	

Soups

canned, dehydrated, and instant soups	bouillon cubes

Packaged foods

processed dinner mixes (e.g., Hamburger Helper, Tuna Twist, Oodles of Noodles, etc.)	packaged gravies, sauces, soups, and seasoning mixes
canned ravioli, spaghetti	TV dinners

Other

baking powder and baking soda	seasoning salts (garlic, onion, lemon, pepper)
meat tenderizers	
Accent	salad dressing
monosodium glutamate (MSG)	pickles
worcestershire sauce	peanut butter
A-1 sauce	sauerkraut
barbecue sauce	catsup
salt	mustard
sea salt	soy sauce
salted snack foods (e.g., potato chips, corn chips, pretzels, popcorn, crackers, nuts)	regular canned vegetables
olives	frozen vegetables with seasoned or cream sauce

sential to proper contraction of muscle (including the heart) as well as being an important substance within virtually all body cells. When the kidneys are incapable of regulating the correct amount of potassium in the body, the ingestion of foods containing large amounts of this mineral must be controlled. Foods generally high in potassium include milk, yogurt, certain fruits and vegetables, whole grains, dried beans, nuts, chocolate, and salt substitutes. Some of the specific foods containing relatively large amounts of potassium are listed in Table 4.

Table 4. Foods and beverages high in potassium

Fruits and juices

apricots	orange juice
avocados	oranges
bananas ˙	persimmons
casaba melons	prune juice
dried fruits	pumpkin
honeydew melons	rhubarb
mangoes	watermelon

Vegetables

artichokes	mustard greens
bamboo shoots	spinach
beet greens	zucchini
broccoli	potato chips
collards	lentils
cress	tomato juice
parsnips	split peas
potatoes	black-eyed peas
raw carrots	beans (white, kidney, black, lima,
raw celery	soy, garbanzo)
squash	brussels sprouts
swiss chard	broccoli
tomato (sauce and paste)	sweet potatoes/yams
tomatoes	water chestnuts

Meats, fish, and poultry*
all

Dairy products*

milk (all types)	custard
yogurt	pudding

Other

bran, bran cereals	coconut
unsweetened baking chocolate	molasses
and cocoa	salt substitutes (potassium chloride)
nuts	

*These foods are basic components of the diets of most people. When your diet is restricted for potassium, you may have these foods, but in limited quantities.

Phosphorus

Phosphorus is a mineral that, along with calcium, is important for normal bone growth and strength. It is common for
the balance of phosphorus and calcium to become disturbed
when kidney function declines; calcium usually is too low

and phosphorus too high. Calcium supplements are prescribed in many cases. However, it is also necessary to decrease the phosphorus in the body to more normal levels.
This control of phosphorus is most often accomplished by a
combination of medication and diet. Foods containing excessive amounts of phosphorus may have to be avoided. Foods
containing relatively high amounts of phosphorus include
milk, yogurt, ice cream, cheese, whole grains, dried beans,
meat, fish, and poultry. Although it is generally impossible
to avoid all such foods while still eating a balanced diet, it is
frequently necessary to limit the amounts, depending upon
the age of the patient and how well medication is working. A
more complete listing of high-phosphorus foods is presented
in Table 5.

Protein

Proteins are the building blocks of all body cells. They are
necessary to keep body tissue in good health, to replace body
cells normally lost each day, and to help us grow normally.

Proteins have their own building blocks called amino acids. There are 21 amino acids. Although the body can manufacture some of these, nine of them must be obtained from
the food we eat. These nine amino acids are referred to as the
essential amino acids. Foods that contain all of the essential
amino acids are called high biological value protein foods.
High biological protein generally comes from animal sources:
poultry, fish, beef, cheese, eggs, and milk are all good
sources. Low biological value protein foods come from
plants: breads, cereals, pasta, rice, and vegetables are all examples of this class of protein. About two-thirds of the protein we eat during the day should be high biological value
protein.

In general, most Americans eat more protein than they actually need. Although this is probably of little consequence
to the normal individual, excessive dietary protein in someone with decreased kidney function may worsen many of the

Table 5. Foods high in phosphorus

Vegetables and fruits

artichokes	lentils
asparagus	avocados
dried beans (kidney, pinto,	broccoli
navy, etc.)	mushrooms
lima beans	brussels sprouts
split peas	peas
vegetables in cream or cheese sauce	

Meat, fish, and poultry

All of these foods are high in phosphorus. Typically, they are not totally eliminated when phosphorus is restricted, but are eaten in limited quantities.

Dairy products

milk, all types	custard
cream	ice cream
yogurt	ice milk
pudding	cheese (except cream and cottage cheeses)

Breads, cereals, and starches

whole wheat bread	bran cereals
pumpernickel bread	ready-to-eat wheat and oat cereals
corn bread	oatmeal
bulgur	Maypo
quick-cooking Cream of Wheat	pancakes/waffles*

Miscellaneous

cream soups	nuts
bean, pea, or split pea soups	cola beverages**
chocolate	

*The phosphorus content of these foods can be decreased by substituting water for at least part of the milk.

**As a rule of thumb, cola beverages contain approximately 50 mg of phosphorus per 12 ounces. This is not a particularly excessive amount, but the clear or fruit-flavored sodas contain little or no phosphorus, making them a better choice.

biochemical disturbances. Many physicians feel that some limitation of dietary protein is useful in managing moderate to severe degrees of kidney failure, although this must be balanced against the protein needs of growing children. Since most high-protein foods are also high in phosphorus, protein limitation also will reduce the intake of phosphorus.

If your child's physician feels that a protein and/or phosphorus restriction will be helpful, guidelines will be provided as to the amount and types of protein to be included in the diet. To follow these guidelines accurately, you will need to see a dietitian to assist you in making the appropriate changes in the amount of protein, in selecting the appropriate balance of high and low biological value protein, and in recommending special low-protein food products, if necessary. The dietitian can also provide you with the names of companies whose products can be purchased and assist you in working them into your meal plan.

Finally, going shopping can become a confusing and frustrating task when you are trying to purchase foods for a special diet. Learning to understand the nutrition information on food labels is one of the first steps in making appropriate food choices to meet the diet needs. Merely reading the labels on food products can be overwhelming for the average shopper, since there is so much information to interpret. In order to give some help, we have provided a sample food label in Figure 28 with some label-reading tips. These pointers emphasize those nutrients that are of particular importance in people with kidney disease.

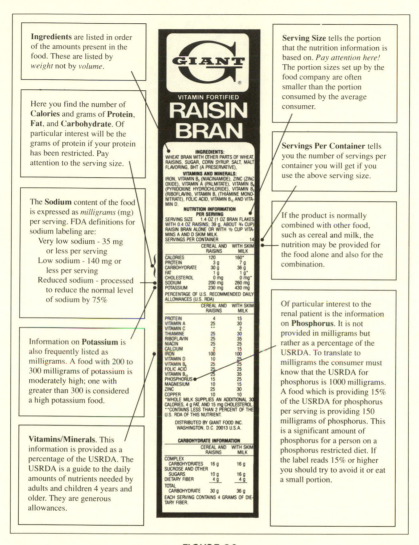

Ingredients are listed in order of the amounts present in the food. These are listed by *weight* not by *volume*.

Here you find the number of **Calories** and grams of **Protein**, **Fat**, and **Carbohydrate**. Of particular interest will be the grams of protein if your protein has been restricted. Pay attention to the serving size.

The **Sodium** content of the food is expressed as *milligrams* (mg) per serving. FDA definitions for sodium labeling are:
Very low sodium - 35 mg or less per serving
Low sodium - 140 mg or less per serving
Reduced sodium - processed to reduce the normal level of sodium by 75%

Information on **Potassium** is also frequently listed as milligrams. A food with 200 to 300 milligrams of potassium is moderately high; one with greater than 300 is considered a high potassium food.

Vitamins/Minerals. This information is provided as a percentage of the USRDA. The USRDA is a guide to the daily amounts of nutrients needed by adults and children 4 years and older. They are generous allowances.

Serving Size tells the portion that the nutrition information is based on. *Pay attention here!* The portion sizes set up by the food company are often smaller than the portion consumed by the average consumer.

Servings Per Container tells you the number of servings per container you will get if you use the above serving size.

If the product is normally combined with other food, such as cereal and milk, the nutrition may be provided for the food alone and also for the combination.

Of particular interest to the renal patient is the information on **Phosphorus**. It is not provided in milligrams but rather as a percentage of the USRDA. To translate to milligrams the consumer must know that the USRDA for phosphorus is 1000 milligrams. A food which is providing 15% of the USRDA for phosphorus per serving is providing 150 milligrams of phosphorus. This is a significant amount of phosphorus for a person on a phosphorus restricted diet. If the label reads 15% or higher you should try to avoid it or eat a small portion.

FIGURE 28

Some useful pointers about the nutritional information contained in a typical product label.

Chapter 8
Psychological Aspects of Chronic Illness in Childhood and Adolescence

The stresses of chronic illness on both the patient and the family can be considerable. These stresses commonly affect self-image, peer and family relationships, school performance, and general quality of life. If medical care is to be complete, it therefore seems senseless to treat the medical illness without also treating the psychological impact of that illness on the patient and family. In order to broaden our perspective in this chapter, we have had the assistance of our pediatric nephrology social worker, Melissa Brown. Missy and her counterparts in other hospitals are very aware of the many nonmedical problems associated with illness, problems that occur regularly and recurrently.

Even the most well adjusted individual may have a significant problem adjusting to having a chronic illness. This is particularly true for children and adolescents who have one of the kidney disorders discussed in previous chapters. These medical problems often cause changes in the appearance of the body, loss of energy, uncertainty about the future, and time away from peers and family. These are major changes for young people, and they are quite likely to affect mental health.

It is not possible to present, in this single chapter, the many aspects of the psychological effects of chronic illness. We will, however, highlight the broad aspects of this problem, drawing from our experience with many patients and families. We suggest that you use this information to be more aware of the problems that might affect your child, your family, or you. In order to be treated, a problem must first be recognized and then be accepted. Since many small problems may grow into large ones, it is important to seek help early, before major difficulties arise. If you think you might benefit from an expert opinion on what to do, request a discussion with the social worker, psychologist, or psychiatrist affiliated with the kidney disease program at your hospital. Remember that the ultimate goal is to improve the quality of life for your entire family and maximize the potential for the affected member of the family.

The Child's Reaction to Illness

It is always a great temptation for parents and health professionals to nurture and protect the young child. In the case of a chronic and potentially serious illness, we have often seen "bad news" withheld from the child because parents felt he or she would have limited understanding of the problem. Withholding information from the child does not prevent anxiety or fear. On the contrary, it may increase these problems. This is particularly true when children are subjected to medical evaluation and treatment and sense their parents' distress without understanding why.

Much of a child's reaction to illness will be based on knowledge of the problem and trust in the medical environment. Although the explanation given should be tailored to the particular child's intellectual and developmental abilities, it is important for your child to believe that he or she is hearing the truth. Make the explanation honest and simple; it is never appropriate to lie. This is an important step in creating a trusting environment for your child—an environment that includes parents and siblings as well as the medical staff. The doctors can often be helpful, since they have had the experience of explaining complicated information in simple terms to many youngsters.

It is difficult to predict how any child will react to having a chronic illness; all children reflect their own personality as well as their environment and family background. Regardless of how the child reacts, it is often reflected in behavior at home, interaction with siblings and peers, and school performance and behavior. Fear, anger, embarrassment, guilt, withdrawal, and depression are all common reactions among children with chronic illnesses. However, children often will not or cannot express these feelings directly. Rather, they may be expressed indirectly at home, in school, or in some other environment in which the child feels more secure. These feelings are often displayed in changes of behavior, such as acting out, poorer school performance, or fighting.

Parents and trusted others can encourage the child to discuss these feelings. These adults—and sometimes older siblings—can acknowledge the fears and place any possible misconceptions in a realistic context. For instance, the child with a chronic but not particularly serious illness may unrealistically fear dying from the disease. It is important to discuss these feelings as soon as possible, so that a pattern of honesty and trust is established with the child, providing the encouragement and security that he or she may need. It is equally important to keep members of the medical team informed of these problems so they may advise and assist in problem-solving.

Also important is the child's need to feel "normal." The inability to participate in some sports or physical activities, a difference in appearance or diet, or having to take some medication at school may be embarrassing and make the child feel different from the other kids. It is normal for a child to be sensitive to these things. This embarrassment may be further increased by reactions from other children or adults who may not completely understand the child's condition. For instance, the child with a kidney abnormality requiring frequent emptying of the bladder can suffer humiliation at the hands of classmates because of those frequent bathroom trips. By explaining your child's illness to teachers, other parents, and other children, you may be able to alleviate or prevent any negative reactions.

The Adolescent's Reaction to Illness

Many important developmental events occur during adolescence. During this time, the teenager is attempting to develop personal independence from the family, learning to fit in with peer groups, and developing interests that may be lifelong (for example, sports, academics, and special talents). Based on this, it should not be surprising that a chronic illness may have a profound effect on a teenager. This may be particularly true when medical care requires time away from peer groups, or if the medical treatment causes physical changes that embarrass the teenager.

In addition to feeling anger, fear, depression, or anxiety, the adolescent patient may also deny the reality of the medical illness, often regardless of the seriousness of the situation. This may be particularly easy for the patient to do when the actual symptoms are minimal. For example, one of our 17-year-old patients had severe hypertension and was at risk for having a seizure or stroke. However, since he felt good at the time, he found no reason to take his blood pressure medicine regularly. He did eventually have a seizure. We counseled him during the hospitalization and hoped that the episode would convince him to comply with the treatment program. Unfortunately, once he left the hospital and felt good again, he went back to his old habits.

As another example, we took care of an attractive and popular high school girl who had a serious form of nephritis. She was initially compliant with her steroid medication until she began to gain weight and develop some acne. She immediately stopped the medication despite a thorough understanding of why this treatment was important. Fortunately, she was able to discuss her fears of the physical changes with her parents and the medical staff, who jointly agreed to "get off her back" and give her a chance to take responsibility for the treatment program. In this case, she successfully got back on track.

Parents of a teenager should keep in mind that when adolescence and chronic illness occur at the same time, it is necessary to separate behavior that may be a result of illness from that which may be regarded as typical of a normal adolescent. As parents of teenagers are well aware, it is often difficult just to understand normal teenage behavior. If behavior is a concern to parents, it is wise to relay these concerns to the social worker, nurse, or physician. They can provide assistance in locating the proper resources for evaluation of the problem and ongoing counseling or advice if needed.

The Effect of Illness on the Family

Regardless of whether it is a child or a teenager who develops the medical problem, the occurrence of a chronic illness will have a tremendous impact on the family. It can affect the parents' marriage, the siblings' relationship with one another, and the quality of family life in general.

Regardless of how the family is affected, the parents often bear much of the initial emotional impact of having a sick child. Parents may initially react to the news with shock or disbelief. They may also feel angry at the medical staff, the child, God, or themselves for the condition of their child. They may resent other parents or other children for having a normal family life. A parent may also feel a great deal of guilt. This may result from a feeling of responsibility for the child's condition or the feeling of helplessness in being unable to control or prevent what has happened. In this situation, parents must guard against the temptation to expend large amounts of energy futilely searching for a cause of the illness. Parents also may feel guilty when having fun or experiencing any happiness at all, knowing that their child is sick.

Parents often direct their anger and resentment toward the medical staff. This often is the result of the increased dependency that they and their child have on other people, making them feel some loss of control over a part of their lives. As a result, parents may behave as if they must manage and control all possible aspects of their child's illness, often ignoring their own needs for relaxation, fun, or relief from the constant pressure. This lack of "down time" can quickly lead to parent burnout, diminished ability to cope with the demands placed on them, and more anger and guilt. We have seen this vicious circle so often that many of us will insist that parents "take a break" when they show the early warning signs of fatigue.

All of these reactions by parents should be considered normal; many parents experience some, if not all, of these feelings at one time or another. There are a number of things that parents can do in order to care for themselves while caring for their child throughout the course of the illness. These are commonsense activities, including eating and exercising regularly, getting sufficient amounts of rest, and ensuring themselves some regular personal time.

There can also be a tremendous benefit from talking to other parents, especially those who have children with similar illnesses or treatments. Many hospitals have support groups for parents of children with various serious illnesses. In these, parents have the opportunity to share information, resources, and concerns. At our hospital, a nephrology parent support group has met monthly for the past three years. We have certain "regulars," and other parents who come and go. Our social workers have tried very hard over the years to encourage parents to attend the meetings. When we ask the parents about this, they often tell us that although it is difficult to motivate themselves to make "yet another trip to the hospital" when it is not medically necessary, they are rarely sorry they attend. This is fairly typical for both parent and patient support groups—they require a lot of energy to maintain but can be very worthwhile for the participants.

The brothers and sisters of the sick child are not exempt from the effects of the illness. They also may experience fear—both for their sibling and from lack of understanding of the disease. In much the same way that the patient needs to have the illness honestly and clearly explained by the doctor or parents, brothers and sisters need similar explanations. In this way, they feel involved, the mystery of the illness can be diminished, and in some cases they can be

reassured of not developing a similar illness. It is also important for parents to be sensitive to the other needs of brothers
and sisters. When the demands of the patient's problems are
considerable, siblings may suffer from lack of attention or
time with their mother and father. This may result in anger
or resentment on the parts of brothers and sisters whose limited understanding makes them view the illness as a way
that the patient gets their parents' attention.

Sibling resentment may also come from inconsistent pa-
rental discipline. Parents often feel guilty when they scold or
punish a child with a medical problem. It may be helpful to
remember that the ultimate goal of discipline is to assist the
child in learning to control and feel responsible for his or her
behavior. By setting limits in a loving but firm manner, the
parent will provide the child with a feeling of security and
reassurance, not punishment; too much freedom can make a
child feel insecure and frightened. Consistency of discipline
is important not only within the family, but from other
adults as well. It may help to discuss this issue with grand-
parents, teachers, and the hospital staff to ensure that your
children are disciplined in a consistent manner.

How the family reacts to the child's illness will depend
upon a variety of factors, largely because people react differently to illness and stress. Some families become stronger
and closer by pulling together during times of crisis, and others benefit from outside resources to help them build communication and support systems at home. The most important step in the process is to ask for the advice of a member of
the medical team in finding the assistance that is most likely
to be of benefit. The ultimate goal is to strike a balance between the needs dictated by the child's illness and those of
the other family members. In this way, the family often can
build on its strengths to meet and overcome emotional challenges.

Chapter 9
A Guide to
Medications

Parents must deal with many potential problems when a child has a kidney disorder. Of these, the difficulties in managing medical therapy can be among the most troublesome. The doctors and other members of your health care team can give you valuable information about your child's specific treatment program. Sometimes, however, it is only through trial and error that parents learn helpful hints, general rules of thumb, and basic drug facts. With the assistance of one of our pediatric nephrology nurse practitioners, Betsy Nicolli, we have gathered information about a variety of medication topics that we think will be of great practical value.

Good Practices for Giving Medication

Many children with kidney disorders must take many medications for long periods of time. Parents often must deal with the very young child who doesn't like their taste or with the older child who just doesn't want to take them. These problems, and many like them, can result in a daily battle between parent and child. There are, fortunately, some tricks (taught to us by parents and patients) for minimizing the struggle.

Establish a Routine

Many of the treatment programs are complex and de-

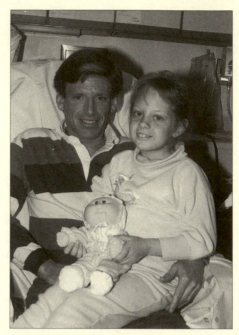

FIGURE 29
The taking of medications can become a major source of conflict between parent and child. Most often, however, reasonable compromises can be found which make medication taking a less stressful occasion for everyone.

manding for the patient as well as the parent. Often, the approach to follow a medication program successfully is similar to that used to teach good general behavior, particularly in young children. This uses the principles of consistency and firmness, while involving the child in decision making.

1. First, establish a routine. If the schedule for taking medication is confusing to you, you can be sure it will be confusing to your child. Therefore, pick specific and reasonable times to give the medications and stick to them as closely as is practical.

2. There are several techniques that can help you and your child remember which medications are taken on which days and at what times. Just having a group of medica-

tion bottles on a shelf will often not do. Pill boxes may be used. These are divided into compartments that can be labeled for different days and times. It is often convenient to "load" them once a week. Medication check-off sheets or calendars may also be hung on the medicine cabinet or refrigerator door to remind you what medications are to be taken on a particular day.

3. Some children will cooperate better with their treatment program if they are allowed to participate in preparing and taking their own medication. Use good judgment in assigning responsibility for taking medication.

4. The bottom line as far as medication is concerned is that you cannot give in if there is resistance to taking it. Your child must learn that the medications taken for kidney disease are necessary and must become part of the daily routine, just like brushing teeth and getting dressed. The sooner this fact is accepted, the sooner battles over medication will end.

5. Review your child's medication list, frequency, and doses with the medical or nursing staff on a regular basis. If you have questions about the purpose or side effects of a particular drug, be sure to ask them. If you are having difficulty purchasing a medication, or are frequently running out, let the physician know. Also, ask about the possibility of simplifying medication schedules.

Look for Practical Solutions

Many medications are not available in a form that is convenient or practical for many infants and children. For instance, the dose in a single tablet or capsule may be too high, the tablet or capsule cannot be swallowed, or a particular medication has a bitter taste that makes it difficult for even a well-intentioned child to take. There are ways to solve these and other problems. While some helpful hints for specific medications are described later in this chapter, there are some general approaches as well. When considering these approaches, it is essential that you check with your doctor first, since it may be improper to use certain techniques for certain medications.

1. The doses of many liquid medications taken by small children and infants are small and difficult to measure. Accuracy may be accomplished best by obtaining a supply of oral syringes (without needles), drawing the solution into the syringe, and then squirting it into the child's mouth. Whenever medication is squirted into the mouth, it should be directed to the side and not toward the back of the throat. This will decrease the risk of choking. Medications specifically designed for children can also be a problem. For example, some are prepared so that the proper dose is a "teaspoon." There is tremendous variability in the volume that a simple teaspoon in the kitchen drawer at home may hold. Therefore, to make sure of a proper dose, you can use a measuring teaspoon, plastic medication cup, or oral syringe marked for the proper volume (one teaspoon is equal to 5 milliliters, often marked as 5 cc or 5 ml). Ask your pharmacist about bottle adapters, which allow for quick and easy withdrawal of liquid medication from the bottle.

2. Some medications come in tablet or capsule form and require other modifications. While there are ways to solve this problem, it is essential to first check with your physician or pharmacist to determine if a particular medication can be given in a more convenient way. This is because some medications cannot or should not be mixed with particular foods or liquids. Many medications can be crushed and mixed with such foods as applesauce, peanut butter, pudding, ice cream, jelly, or yogurt to be fed to young children or babies. Remember to mix the medication in a small spoonful of these foods to assure that the child receives the full dose. Alternatively, some juices may hide the bitter taste of certain medications. Care must be taken if you use one of your child's favorite foods, however, since he or she might resent altering the taste and begin to refuse foods or formula that are needed for proper nutrition.

Anticipate Problems

The importance of taking prescribed medication accurately should be obvious. Even if this occurs, there are some situations that can result in other problems. Recognizing these can prevent unnecessary difficulties.

1. It is not advisable to give a child with kidney disease over-the-counter (nonprescription) medications or home remedies that have not been prescribed or approved by your physician. First, potentially harmful interactions can occur between your child's regular medicines and other medications. Also, some common remedies can have serious side effects in a child with kidney disease that would not ordinarily happen to a healthy child. Finally, some home remedies that seem innocent can have substances that are not handled well in someone whose kidney function is not normal. Therefore, it is always wise to consult the physician first before giving your child such things as vitamins, cold medicines, aspirin, so-called non-aspirin pain medications, cough syrup, laxatives, and other common medications or home remedies.

2. Be sure to keep your pediatrician informed of the names of all medications your child is taking for the kidney disease. Your child's pediatrician may find it necessary to prescribe other treatments from time to time, such as antibiotics or routine immunizations. Even these types of treatments must take into consideration such factors as other medications as well as the child's current medical condition.

3. Keep track of medication supplies. This also includes making sure that you have enough medication to last through weekends and holidays as well as during vacations. If an extended trip is planned, you might carry an extra prescription for essential medications in your wallet. In this way you can be prepared for unexpected situations, such as if the medication is misplaced or the airline loses your baggage.

4. If your child is receiving some form of dialysis, it may become necessary to adjust the timing of the dose around the dialysis treatment schedule, because some medications are affected by dialysis.
5. Remember that even though your child needs medications, they could be very dangerous to other family members. KEEP ALL MEDICATIONS OUT OF THE REACH OF CHILDREN.
6. Medications generally should be stored in a cool, dry location. Storage in a bathroom medicine cabinet must often be avoided because of frequent heat and moisture.

General Hints for Medication Purchase

Pharmacists place a professional emphasis on providing you with a carefully prepared and accurate prescription drug for your child. However, here are some guidelines you can follow in obtaining high-quality and cost-saving pharmacy services.

1. Get to know your pharmacists. Let them know that your child has a particular medical condition. If the pharmacy has the ability to keep a list of your child's medications on a computer, take advantage of this free service. Keep this computer list up to date on all medications and doses, and request computer screening for undesirable drug interactions when new medications are prescribed.
2. Many medications come in tablet or capsule dosage forms unsuitable for children. Although mixing "parts" of tablets or capsules in food is often a practical solution, as described earlier, some medications cannot or should not be mixed. Your pharmacist can investigate individual medications to determine whether certain drugs can be specially prepared in liquid form. There is often a separate charge for this service, but the convenience and accuracy are worthwhile.

3. When filling a prescription, ask your pharmacist how the medication is supplied by the manufacturer. Often, a bottle of medication can be purchased as it comes from the supplier. You then can avoid being charged for the pharmacist to dispense a smaller number of pills than was contained in the original bottle.

4. Many insurance companies provide some coverage for medication costs. If yours does so, check to see if you can order your prescriptions through a contract pharmacy. This type of pharmacy often provides fast service with telephone ordering, home delivery, and direct billing to your insurance company.

5. When having prescriptions filled, do not allow the pharmacist to substitute an alternate drug without first consulting with your physician.

6. Whenever a new medication is prescribed, be sure to remind the pharmacist and the physician of any medication allergies your child may have. Many people with specific drug allergies can have similar reactions to related drug compounds.

7. Ask your physician about prescribing generic rather than brand name medications.

Antihypertensive Medications

As we have discussed in previous chapters, high blood pressure (hypertension) is common in children with kidney disease. An excessively high blood pressure can lead to serious damage to many internal organs such as the brain and heart. In addition, a great deal of research has shown that even modestly elevated blood pressure can increase the rate at which diseased kidneys deteriorate. Therefore, there are several good reasons to take the treatment of high blood pressure seriously.

It may be difficult to motivate older children and young adults to take their blood pressure medication regularly. This is undoubtedly at least partly because many people with hy-

pertension feel no symptoms. It is difficult to motivate someone to take medicine for a problem that doesn't make them
feel bad.

Many physicians will first resort to certain dietary restrictions when attempting to reduce blood pressure (see chapter 7). Your physician can keep you up to date on many of
the new approaches to dietary control of blood pressure.
When diet alone is not enough to keep the blood pressure at
an acceptable level, medication is often prescribed. This
group of drugs is collectively called "antihypertensive medication."

You will recall from earlier chapters that blood pressure is
increased through a combination of two forces: increasing
the amount of fluid (and accompanying salt) in the blood
vessels and decreasing the size of the blood vessel itself. Similarly, medications that reduce blood pressure generally do
so either by forcing the body to eliminate extra salt and water
or by relaxing the muscles in the walls of the blood vessels
and thereby increasing their size. How each type of medication actually accomplishes this varies tremendously. Although water balance and the kidney hormone, renin, play
important roles in altering blood pressure, they interact with
other body forces that affect water balance and blood vessel
muscle tone. These forces include the nervous system and
other substances that cause blood vessels to narrow or to
relax. The fact that different medications affect these systems
in a variety of ways gives the physician the ability to more
effectively tailor treatment to the individual needs of the
patient.

Finally, if your child has a significant problem with hypertension, we suggest that you ask the doctor about obtaining
a blood pressure cuff and stethoscope so you can learn
to take the blood pressure yourself. Most parents and adolescents can be trained to perform this task accurately in a
single short session. Home blood pressure readings are a
great help in making proper treatment decisions. First of
all, there are times when the anxiety of visiting the hospital or doctor's office is enough temporarily to raise the
blood pressure. Comparing office readings to those from

home can help in determining if the blood pressure is too high too much of the time. Also, many antihypertensive medications have variable effects on different individuals. For example, if your child gets a single dose of a blood pressure medicine each morning, and the blood pressure is always normal during that early afternoon clinic visit, what about in the evening, or first thing in the morning? Reporting the results of blood pressure recordings from various times during the day and night from home is better than running to the nurse several times a day.

Alternatively, many physicians now have blood pressure recorders that your child can "wear" for 24 hours. These devices will automatically take and record the blood pressure during the day and during sleep so that the consistency of blood pressure control can be determined.

What follows is a basic discussion of the major classes of antihypertensive medications. New drugs are being developed at an ever-increasing rate. Therefore, although this and the following sections provide general drug information, ask your doctor or pharmacist to provide you with the most up-to-date details.

Diuretics

Action

The diuretics are a group of drugs that increase salt and water elimination by the kidneys. This reduces the volume of fluid in the body and thus lowers blood pressure. In certain forms of hypertension, diuretics alone can be effective. They are also commonly used in combination with other antihypertensive medications, however. In these situations, the effect of one medication complements the other to afford good blood pressure control.

Several different classes of diuretics exist, each causing increased salt and water excretion in a different manner. Rather than going into detail about each drug, each class will be generally described as will some possible side effects and helpful hints as to their use. Only the generic (chemical) name of medications will be used since many

different brand names often exist for each specific com-
pound.

Thiazides

Examples: Chlorothiazide, hydrochlorothiazide, metola-
zone.
Side effects: Dry mouth, thirst, weakness, drowsiness or
restlessness, diarrhea or upset stomach, dizziness or lightheadedness when getting up from a lying or sitting position;
potassium loss that can cause hypokalemia, which means an
abnormally low level of potassium in the blood. Hypokalemia is a common and important complication of many types
of diuretics and may require extra dietary or supplemental
potassium (see chapter 7). Signs of an excessively low potassium level include muscle pains and cramps, an irregular
heartbeat, a weak pulse, nausea, or vomiting.

Loop diuretics

Examples: Furosemide, ethacrynic acid, bumetanide.
Side effects: See those for thiazides; also oral and gastric
(stomach) burning, muscle cramps, and potassium loss (hypokalemia).

Potassium-sparing diuretic

(This often helps decrease potassium losses caused by other
diuretics.)
Example: Spironolactone.
Side effects: Drowsiness, headache, skin eruptions or hives,
confusion, loss of balance, stomach upset or diarrhea, high
potassium levels (hyperkalemia).

Hints about Diuretics

Since salt in the diet can usually raise blood pressure significantly, most children who are prescribed diuretics to
help control their blood pressure will also be told to follow a
diet low in salt and sodium. This is an essential part of the
treatment because excessive salt intake will defeat the action
of the diuretic. Contact the renal dietitian for advice about
how to put together a reasonable restricted diet. As an aside,

the average adult diet contains many times the amount of salt required each day. Many physicians believe that this excessive salt intake contributes to elevated blood pressures in certain individuals. Since no possible harm can come about from diminishing dietary salt intake in an otherwise normal individual, it would serve the family well (and set a good example at the same time!) if the entire family changed its eating habits.

Also remember that the diuretics may increase the amount or frequency of urination. This is a potential problem in school or at night. Depending on the child's schedule and the schedule of the medication, it might be best to give the medication early in the morning and, if necessary, early in the evening. Check with your doctor before changing any dosage schedule.

In order to evaluate the effectiveness of the diuretic, your physician may ask you to periodically keep daily records of your child's weight, fluid intake, and urine volume.

Beta-blockers

Action

This group of antihypertensive medications has been around for quite a while and is one of the most frequently prescribed. Beta-blockers inhibit certain types of nerve impulses that contribute to maintaining high blood pressure. As a result of quieting this type of nerve signal, the amount of blood being pumped out of the heart can be modestly diminished and blood vessel muscle "tone" decreased at the same time. The result is a decrease in overall blood pressure.

Examples: Atenolol, metoprolol, nadolol, pindolol, propranolol.

Side effects: Decreased heart rate, possible decreased exercise tolerance (since increase of heart rate with exercise may be blocked), dizziness or lightheadedness, possible fluid retention when salt is not restricted, wheezing.

Hints

Never stop these medications without consulting a physician

first. Propranolol is usually discontinued by tapering the dosage. Suddenly discontinuing it may cause a dangerous, exaggerated increase in blood pressure. If your child has had asthma or wheezing in the past, beta-blockers should be selected carefully because some may actually cause potentially severe asthma attacks.

Alpha-blockers

Action

This type of drug also acts on nerves, by blocking the signals to selected nerves causing blood vessel muscles to contract. As a result, the blood vessels relax and the blood pressure falls.

Examples: Prazosin, labetalol (combined alpha and beta blocker).

Side effects: Dizziness and lightheadedness (especially when standing quickly), headache, drowsiness, lethargy, nausea, palpitations. Many of the initial side effects disappear over several days to weeks with continued therapy.

Hint

If taking this medicine, use extra care during exercise or during hot weather or if you must stand for long periods of time.

Central Nervous System Agents

Action

This is another type of medication that acts on nerve signals contributing to maintaining high blood pressure. In this case, the medication acts to change the production of signals from the brain, so that the blood vessels in the body can relax.

Example: Clonidine.

Side effects: Dry mouth, sedation, dizziness, fatigue, constipation, headache, sodium and water retention, insomnia, nightmares.

Hints

To avoid potentially dangerous "rebound" hypertension as described previously for propranolol, the medicine should be discontinued gradually over two to four days. Always keep enough of this medication on hand. Do not run out of medication! This drug can commonly add to the effects of central nervous system depressants (medications that can include antihistamines, sedatives, analgesics, or seizure medications).

Vasodilators

Action

These medications also act to relax the muscles of many blood vessels. In this case, they do so by acting directly on the smooth muscles in the walls of the blood vessels. As blood flow becomes less restricted, blood pressure declines.
Examples: Hydralazine, minoxidil.
Side effects: Hydralazine—headaches, palpitations, loss of appetite, nausea, dizziness, sweating. Minoxidil—fluid retention, increase in the growth of hair on the back, arms, face, legs, and scalp.

Hints

Minoxidil is a very effective medication that can be particularly useful in some patients with severe hypertension. The hair growth is usually an unacceptable side effect in children with kidney disorders. Some parents have successfully used a depilatory (chemical hair remover) to control the excess growth.

"ACE" Inhibitors

Action

"ACE" stands for angiotensin II-converting enzyme (easy to see why we use "ACE"). As we have mentioned, one of the ways the kidney causes blood pressure to rise is via the hormone renin. The most potent portion of the action of renin occurs via the action of ACE. Therefore, this group of drugs causes blood vessels to relax and decreases salt and water retention by blocking the action of ACE. These medications have been an important development in the treatment of high blood pressure.

Examples: Captopril, enalapril, lisinopril, ramipril.

Side effects: Skin rash, dizziness or lightheadedness, drowsiness, hyperkalemia (excessive and potentially dangerous blood level of potassium).

Hints

If drowsiness persists while taking a once-a-day dose, try taking the medicine at bedtime. Avoid taking captopril within one hour of meals since food may decrease the amount of medication absorbed into the body. The rise of blood potassium level may be partly offset by avoiding high-potassium foods (see chapter 7).

Calcium Channel Blockers

Action

Movement of calcium into the muscle cells is essential to the contraction of the muscles of the heart and blood vessels. These medicines interfere with calcium movement into the muscle cells. As a result, the muscles of the heart and blood vessels relax, causing reduction in blood pressure.

Examples: Nifedipine, verapamil.

Side effects: Swelling of ankles, feet or lower legs, dizziness or lightheadedness (especially when moving quickly from a lying to a sitting or standing position), headache (usually resolves once the medicine has been taken for a few weeks).

Hints

Take one hour before or two hours after meals. If you miss a dose, take it as soon as possible. If it is within two hours of the next dose, do not take the missed dose at all and do not double the next one.

Common Chemical Imbalances and Their Treatments

Potassium

Action

Most of the potassium in the body is held inside cells, and the actual concentration of potassium in the blood and fluids outside the cells is closely monitored and maintained by the kidneys. Many people with moderately advanced kidney disease have problems eliminating excess potassium from the body, although in certain types of kidney disorders too much potassium is lost in the urine. Certain medications, particularly most diuretics, may also cause excessive potassium losses.

Why is potassium so important? This mineral is critical in the efficient and proper function of many processes in the body, one of the most important of which is nerve and muscle function. Excessively low or (more commonly) high potassium levels can lead to abnormal muscle function, including the possibility of sudden and potentially fatal heart problems. Therefore, the balance of potassium in the body is taken very seriously. We have already discussed the treatment of low potassium levels in the section about diuretics. Below we discuss the treatment of chronically elevated potassium levels.

Example: Sodium polystyrene sulfonate (Kayexalate).
Side effects: Diarrhea, nausea, fluid retention.

Hints

Kayexalate removes potassium through the intestine by exchanging it for sodium. Therefore, it can add to the body's burden of sodium, worsening fluid retention, swelling, and hypertension. While on this medication, it is wise to pay particular attention to avoiding sodium-containing foods. Chronically elevated potassium levels are uncommon after infancy in patients who are not yet nearing dialysis. Most often, a significant part of the problem is the large amounts of potassium in many favorite foods. Refer to chapter 7 for a list of these high-potassium foods.

Calcium

Action

Like potassium, calcium is a mineral playing an essential role in many body processes. It is essential for the normal growth and strength of bones, is a critical component of a great number of biochemical reactions within cells, and plays an important role in muscle function, including the heart. As previously discussed in chapters 1 and 5, calcium balance in the body is maintained by the delicate and complex balance of hormones (particularly parathyroid hormone and the form of vitamin D activated by the kidney) and the levels of calcium and phosphorus in the blood. It is common for calcium levels to be too low in patients with significant kidney dysfunction, a problem of particular significance to growing children. Very low calcium levels in the blood can cause muscle cramps, convulsions, or irregularities of heart beat. The most common initial approach to this problem is to treat the calcium deficiency with some combination of calcium supplementation and the specialized active forms of vitamin D.

Examples of calcium supplements: Calcium salts (carbonate, glubionate, gluconate).

Side effects: Chalky taste, nausea, constipation, excessively high calcium level.

Examples of "active" vitamin D forms: Dihydrotachysterol (DHT), calcitriol, calcifediol.

Side effects: Constipation, excessively high calcium level (hypercalcemia, which can result from too high an intake of calcium or from overtreatment with vitamin D. Common symptoms and signs of moderate elevations of calcium include increased blood pressure, irritability, diminished appetite, and the deposition of calcium crystals within body tissues, causing tissue damage).

Hints

Foods such as spinach, rhubarb, bran, and whole grain cereals bind calcium in the intestine. An excessive intake of these foods may diminish the effect of supplemental dietary calcium. Calcium carbonate supplements are often used as phosphorus binders (see below) rather than primarily to provide extra calcium. If given as a binder, give with meals. If given as a calcium supplement, give at least one hour after meals to promote calcium absorption. Many patients comment on the bitter taste of calcitriol (Rocaltrol). You usually can get infants and toddlers to take it by squirting it into applesauce. Dihydrotachysterol (DHT) mixes well with orangeade to hide the unusual taste.

Phosphorus

Action

Phosphorus is a mineral found in many foods, particularly those rich in animal or dairy protein. Children with significant kidney disease may be unable to excrete phosphate properly. Its accumulation in the bloodstream can lead to improper bone formation and growth. Phosphate binders are drugs that bind to phosphorus in the bowel and prevent it from being absorbed into the bloodstream. Many antacid medications work well as phosphate binders. These include the aluminum-containing and calcium carbonate antacids (see earlier). When phosphorus combines with aluminum or calcium, an insoluble material is formed and excreted in stool, and thus, not absorbed into the body.
Examples: Calcium carbonate, aluminum hydroxide gel, aluminum carbonate.
Side effects: Constipation, chalky taste, nausea, belching.

Hints

Antacids should be given at least 30 minutes after most other medications as they may interfere with their absorption into the body. Phosphate binders must be given with meals in order to have optimal effects. Liquid calcium carbonate does not mix well with many foods and fluids. If your child prefers, these medications are available in chewable tablets. Most children dislike the chalky taste of these medications. Unfortunately they must accept the taste and learn it is essential that they be taken. There are cookie recipes that can be made with many of the antacids. You may want to ask your dietitian for recipes and other ideas about cooking with these medications.

Acid Imbalance (Acidosis)

Action

Children with significant kidney disease have problems with their acid-base balance. The balancing of acids and bases in the body is critical to the function of most biochemical reactions in the body. The more disturbed the balance, the more inefficient the reactions critical to life. Most of the time, the imbalance results from excess acids, since the kidneys may be unable to appropriately excrete the constantly produced acid waste products of normal metabolism. To maintain the acid-base balance and to make up for the excess acid in the blood, a medicine that provides a base (usually bicarbonate or citrate) is given.

Examples: Sodium bicarbonate, sodium citrate, potassium citrate solutions.

Side effects: Belching, gas or swelling of the stomach, stomach cramps, diarrhea, unusual increase in thirst.

Hints

Chilling the citrate solution (Bicitra or Polycitra) or taking it with water or juice may improve the taste. These medications should generally be given at least one hour after most other medications. Sodium bicarbonate can increase fluid retention and hypertension as a result of its sodium content.

Immunosuppressive Medications

As discussed in previous chapters, several types of kidney problems require medications that act to alter certain aspects of the body's immune system. An unavoidable side effect of the majority of these medications is an impaired ability to respond to natural infections (both bacterial and viral), as well as to immunizations such as the measles and oral polio vaccines. This is a particular problem for young children receiving these drugs, since they are the ones who require many of these immunizations. They are also the ones most frequently exposed to viral infections such as chickenpox and measles.

The most common settings in which these medications are used are in childhood nephrotic syndrome, certain forms of glomerulonephritis, and transplantation. Many of these medications have overlapping effects and can be used in many different combinations. A brief discussion of some of the major immunosuppressive medications in use today follows.

Corticosteroids ("Steroids")

Action

This is a group of steroid hormone medications similar to those made normally by the body. The actual way in which these hormones affect the immune system is not completely understood. We do know that they exert an effect on the function of white blood cells (lymphocytes), which regulate and promote many types of inflammatory reactions. This class of medication is the one most commonly used in "anti-immune" therapy in pediatric nephrology. They are the current mainstay of treatment in childhood nephrotic syndrome, effective in certain forms of nephritis, and a part of most transplant treatment programs.

Examples: Many types of corticosteroids exist. Those most commonly used are prednisone, prednisolone, methylprednisolone.

Side effects: Increased appetite, weight gain, salt and water retention often resulting in swelling and high blood pressure, flushing and facial fullness ("cushingoid facies"), increased soft hair and acne, stomach irritation with possible bleeding, mood swings, increased risk of infection, cataracts, loss of calcium from the bones, skin "stretch" marks.

The risks of most of these possible side effects increase with increasing dose or duration of therapy.

Certain other complications of steroid treatment occur rarely, but should be reported to the physician immediately if they occur: Frequent and severe stomach pain or vomiting, temperature over 102 F, dizziness or weakness, blurring of vision, or any infection other than a cold.

Hints

Take this medicine with meals. If stomach irritation becomes a problem, ask your physician about taking an antacid. Your child may need to be on a salt-restricted diet while on high doses of this medicine. Home monitoring of blood pressure and daily weight may need to be done. It is common for children on high doses of steroids to get an oral yeast infection (thrush). This is a result of the drug's effect on the immune system. Another medicine, called nystatin, is prescribed to be swished in the mouth after meals to treat the thrush.

To help children and teens keep from becoming obese from the steroid treatment, parents often need to set limits on the quantity and types of foods eaten during and between meals. Although many parents are ecstatic to see their kids' appetites return after prolonged illness or after a successful transplant, it is sad to see them develop excessive obesity as a result of treatment. Learning dietary self-control early on can help prevent a lifelong weight problem for children on chronic steroid therapy.

Anyone who has received high doses of steroid medication for more than several weeks should not have the medication suddenly discontinued. Some steroid hormone is essential for body function. With steroid treatment the body finds it unnecessary to produce its own. It takes time for the adrenal gland to again produce its own steroid, which is the reason that most doctors slowly lower (sometimes referred to as "taper"), rather than suddenly stop, these medicines after a prolonged period of therapy.

Azathioprine

Action

This medication produces its effect on the immune system by suppressing the production of rapidly growing and dividing cells. Since white blood cells in the immune system, when stimulated, will enter a rapid growth phase, the drug is an effective inhibitor of immune function.

Side effects: Increased risk of infection, loss of appetite, nausea and vomiting, possible hair thinning, decreased white blood cell count as well as decrease in other blood cells, liver injury.

The following side effects are rare but should be reported to the physician immediately if they occur: fever, chills, sore throat, unusual bleeding or bruising, unusual tiredness or weakness, yellowing of the eyes or skin.

Hint

The medicine should be taken with or directly after meals, as it may cause nausea or vomiting if taken on an empty stomach.

Cyclophosphamide and Chlorambucil

Action

Both of these medications are also beneficial in some immune diseases. They are also used, in certain circumstances, as cancer treatment drugs—a fact mentioned here because it often comes up in discussions with parents. These medications exert their effect by slowing the growth of rapidly dividing cells (see azathioprine). Although these drugs have several uses in the treatment of pediatric kidney disease, they are most frequently used as "second-line" drugs in childhood nephrotic syndrome and in certain forms of nephritis.

Side effects: Both drugs increase the risk of infection and can cause loss of appetite, nausea, vomiting, and liver dysfunction. There is also increased risk of anemia or bleeding, and certain age groups may be at risk for having infertility as

adults. Also, cyclophosphamide can cause transient loss of
hair and severe bladder irritation.

Cyclosporine A

Action

This relatively new and important drug interferes with the
activity of specific lymphocytes that play a crucial role in ac-
tivating the immune system. Unlike many other immunosuppressive medications, cyclosporine does not depress the
function of the bone marrow; thus, other blood cells, even
those with certain immune functions, still may be manufactured. Cyclosporine has had a dramatic effect on the success
rate of transplantation, and it also has potential application
in other diseases.
Side effects: Tremors or slight shaking of the hands, excessive hair growth, high blood pressure, swollen or bleeding
gums, kidney or liver dysfunction.
    The following side effects are extremely rare but should be
reported to the physician immediately if they occur: seizures,
fever or chills, sore throat, persistent vomiting, jaundice (yellowing of the skin or eyes), diminished urination.

Hints

Store the medication in a cool (do not refrigerate) and safe
place away from children. The medicine may be mixed with
milk, chocolate milk, or orange juice to improve its taste. Mix
well and have your child drink the entire amount immediately.

Antibodies

Action

Antibodies (contained in antisera or in purified form) are
substances that can attach very specifically to chemical structures in the body. In the case of transplantation, this class of
substances includes various preparations of antisera or antibodies that are directed against lymphocyte-type cells of the
immune system. Like many other antibody preparations,

they are manufactured through a variety of different methods from different animals (horse, goat, mouse). When these antibodies attach to their "target" (in this case those cells that activate other cells of the immune system), a number of processes occur that ultimately result in destruction of the target. This becomes a very potent method for controlling immune reactions in some serious immune diseases affecting the kidney, such as transplant rejection. However, the effectiveness of these preparations, and the fact that they come from foreign (animal) sources, makes their use feasible for only short courses of therapy.

The antibody OKT3 differs from other antibodies in that it is very specific for the activator immune cells. This makes the preparation not only very effective, but also avoids many of the side effects resulting from previous types of antibodies, which tended to react with other types of cells as well.

Side effects: Fever, chills, rash, and dangerous blood pressure elevation or other allergic type symptoms. Decreased levels of cells other than lymphocytes may lead to increased risk for serious infection or bleeding. The initial reaction to the administration of OKT3 can be quite dramatic, with high fever, chills, diarrhea, headaches, and, rarely, difficulty breathing. These symptoms usually are seen only following the first or second dose and will resolve during the treatment course.

Other

Erythropoietin

Action

Recently the hormone erythropoietin has been synthesized in the laboratory. In healthy people this hormone is made in the kidney and circulates to the bone marrow, where it is essential in controlling the production of red blood cells. Patients with kidney failure often lack adequate amounts of this hormone and thus are anemic. The synthetic hormone now can be given to patients with kidney disease, thereby preventing the need for frequent blood transfusions. The hormone is effective only if it is injected into a vein or under the skin (subcutaneously). It takes several weeks for the anemia to start to improve. Since this hormone stimulates the bone marrow to use iron to make new red blood cells, the amount of iron stored in the body is very important in determining how well a patient will respond. Many patients must take iron supplements for the erythropoietin to work effectively.

Human Growth Hormone

Action

Human growth hormone also has been synthesized recently in the laboratory. This hormone stimulates growth in height in many children and is currently used most often in children who have a deficiency in growth hormone. This hormone is currently being studied in children with renal disease who are very short. It must be given by needle under the skin (subcutaneously) on a frequent basis. It is effective only if given before the child begins puberty. The long-term benefit as well as the side effects currently are being investigated. At the moment it is not generally available.

Chapter 10
What I Wish I Had Known . . .

This chapter presents a potpourri of information. The subjects were selected after talking to many parents who told us what they wished they had known when they began coping with their child's kidney disorder.

In the previous chapters, we presented information about the function of the kidneys, the disorders that may occur and how they are treated, and the psychological effects of disease on the child and family. This chapter will discuss some practical information from which parents might benefit. Having some knowledge of these subjects can ease the hospitalization process, assist in planning finances, and ensure that families take full advantage of available resources. The most important practical tip is to be assertive in finding out what you need to know and do. There is no requirement that parents live in mystery: Ask! If someone doesn't know the answer, then ask who does.

Who's in Charge Here?

Often, a child with a kidney disorder will be referred by the personal physician to the pediatric nephrology subspecialist for assistance in diagnosis or treatment. Many of these subspecialists practice in hospitals affiliated with medical schools, since, in addition to patient care, these doctors also are often involved in medical teaching and/or research. Therefore, a child is often cared for by a group of people, including a variety of health professionals as well as individuals in various phases of their training. Many people are suspicious of these so-called "teaching institutions." They commonly ask questions such as: "Why must we see so many different doctors?" "Why must we see students?" "Will they experiment on my child?" It is important to remember that:

1. Many of the advances used to treat highly complex diseases such as those of the kidney were developed at institutions like these.

2. The manner in which medicine is practiced and the resources available at these types of hospitals are specifically designed to meet the needs of patients with more uncommon types of illnesses.

3. Part of the reason these types of medical centers exist is to support medical school and residency educational programs and university research programs. Some of the financial support for these hospitals comes from these activities, and most of the physicians at these hospitals are committed to these activities. Therefore, your participation in medical education often is expected if you are to take advantage of the teaching hospital's resources.

4. All health professionals conducting any form of human research are first required to seek approval for the research project from an institutional research board. Then, you must be asked and provide written agreement before any research is performed on your child. In most medical centers, only a small fraction of patients actually participate in research projects. If you are asked to take part in such a program, you may ask any questions you have before deciding whether you agree to have yourself and/or your child participate.

On one hand, much of the current knowledge about diseases such as those of the kidney is a result of human research having been performed in the past. Likewise, future progress depends upon current research. On the other hand, if you choose not to participate and you continue to receive care in the same institution, the medical staff is required to provide the same quality of care you would have received as a participant in a research program.

In addition to these issues, parents and patients often become confused by the sheer number and titles of the people caring for them. Described below are several types of health professionals with whom you may come in contact in a pediatric kidney disease program.

Your child's attending physician is the member of the medical staff at the hospital who is ultimately responsible for the care given your child. This physician may be assisted by a variety of other health care professionals, including other physicians. However, he or she is the top banana for your child's case. Depending on the workings of any particular hospital, the attending physician may be the nephrologist caring for your child or another physician for whom the nephrologist is the consultant (see below).

A consultant may be another physician or a different type of health care professional. The consultant is generally an individual who is an expert in a particular field (just like the pediatric nephrologist is an expert in children's kidney diseases). In situations where the opinions or abilities of several different medical specialists are required, your attending physician may request the assistance of several consultants.

The pediatric nephrology fellow is a physician who often works with the nephrologist. This individual is a fully trained and qualified pediatrician who has decided to spend an additional two or three years studying the field of children's kidney disease in order to become a certified expert in kidney diseases of childhood. The fellow often assists the nephrologist with much of the day-to-day medical care in the hospital.

The pediatric resident is a physician who, after completing medical school, has decided to become a pediatric specialist. In most places, this requires three years of further training in the field of pediatrics under the supervision of pediatric attending physicians, including the pediatric nephrologist.

Medical students spend the latter two years of their medical school training learning patient care under the supervision of the physicians at the hospital. It is only through direct patient care that the students can develop the skills and much of the knowledge they will need to become independent and highly qualified physicians.

The staffs of many hospitals and physician's offices have been joined by nurse practitioners. These are individuals who have completed their undergraduate nursing degrees (RNs), have had experience in patient care, and have returned to school to receive further training and an advanced degree in physical diagnosis and patient care. Nurse practitioners may have specialty areas much like many physicians. Thus, a nurse practitioner may work with the pediatric nephrologist in daily patient care activities and is often also responsible for a variety of patient and parent educational programs in many institutions.

Although the individuals listed above are only a small portion of the health professionals you may encounter, they are the ones about whose roles parents most often become confused.

Patients' Rights and Responsibilities

In order to assist patients and their families in understanding their rights while receiving medical care, most hospitals have copies of these rights available upon request. The next paragraph includes several of these generally accepted rights, which are of fundamental importance. You may request the complete list at your hospital.

All patients and their guardians have the right to participate in the planning of the medical treatment and, as mentioned above, have the right to refuse to participate in medical research. Patients and guardians also have the right to review their medical record, although the manner in which this may occur varies from institution to institution. They also must receive, upon request, information about other medical facilities available to them. Finally, parents have the right to express their concerns, grievances, and recommendations to the staff. Many hospitals now have patient representatives, whose primary job is to assist patients and parents in resolving questions or problems that might arise during the course of medical care.

While these "consumer" rights may be freely exercised by all patients and parents, many are hesitant to do so. Presumedly, this is out of the concern that they will anger the staff and that the quality of care will suffer. Most health professionals truly aspire to provide excellence in care and feel it is important that they are made aware of problems. The potential benefits to be derived from expressing a problem or particular dissatisfaction far outweighs the unlikely negative reaction of a particular health professional.

Second Opinions

When parents have doubts about a diagnosis, recommended treatment, or surgical procedure, a second opinion may be appropriate. Few physicians are offended by this request, and they often feel second opinions provide reassurance and ultimately strengthen their relationship with the family and patient. Therefore, most pediatric nephrologists will assist your search for an equally qualified subspecialist from whom a second opinion can be sought.

Obtaining the opinion of a second physician can be reassuring. Be cautious of several potential pitfalls, however. It is in your best interest to be honest with your physician about your intent to consult another. If you decide to return to the first doctor after getting the second opinion, there is a much greater likelihood of creating mistrust from a "behind-the-back" second opinion than of causing anger from honesty. Another reason for being up front with your doctor is that you can easily obtain a copy of the medical record. In the situation where a family comes for a second opinion without previous written information, the quality and accuracy of the second opinion are jeopardized and the process of reevaluation may be redundant, expensive, and prolonged.

Finally, carefully examine the reasons you desire a second opinion. These opinions can be useful in the process of seeking the best medical care available. However, we have seen some families go to excess, often at great expense, almost as if they are unconsciously searching for a different or more favorable medical judgment. Often your family physician can help you determine whether the second opinion you seek is a sensible and worthwhile one or not.

Education During Illness

As a result of certain types of kidney diseases, a child or adolescent can miss a great deal of school. For instance, a child with a recurring or chronic illness may have frequent clinical appointments and insufficient energy to keep up the pace that daily school activities require. Or, the adolescent requiring hemodialysis misses a great deal of school while getting treatments two or three times a week.

Public law 94-142, passed in 1975, addresses the public school responsibilities in these types of situations. Essentially, this law states that children with serious medical conditions or handicaps have the same right to an education as any other child. What this means is that the school authorities in your home town are required to work with you on finding a way to continue your child's education even if he or she is unable to attend school regularly. The specific regulations vary in different school jurisdictions, as do the options. While a particular school district may make greater use of home tutors for children unable to attend school regularly, another might employ remedial study programs. Regardless, the teachers and principals are required to help your child keep up with the school programs.

If you feel your child is entitled to and may benefit from some form of supplemental educational program, first check with the school to find out what type of information is required. Frequently, you must provide some form of doctor's statement detailing the reasons your child is unable to attend school regularly. The doctor might also have to provide some of the medical details that have caused the problem. Many hospitals have social workers or educational counselors who can help you with this process by providing advice as to whether the child falls into a category of eligibility and assisting in locating various resources in the school system that can best meet your child's needs.

Health Insurance and Medical Costs

The medical costs associated with a major illness can be considerable, sometimes financially devastating a family. That is why it is so important to be sure that your family maintains a reasonable level of health insurance. Even if you have done so, a thorough understanding of the details of your insurance coverage and help with financial planning are very important. Insurance reimbursement can become extremely confusing, especially in some situations with kidney disease. As a result, many hospitals have credit or business offices that can provide a number of services to you and your family. Financial counselors there can help you understand your policy and the procedures you must follow to receive insurance reimbursement. They often can work out a payment program for the uninsured balance, which can take into consideration the family's financial situation.

It is important that you anticipate insurance and payment problems. We have heard many stories from families who did not follow proper procedure as outlined in their insurance contracts. As a result, the insurance company had the right to refuse payment. For example, many insurance companies require that you obtain preauthorization for admission to the hospital for an "elective" (non-emergency) procedure. If you do not obtain this preauthorization from your insurer in writing, they have the right to refuse to pay, even if the hospitalization was technically covered by your policy.

In addition, many health insurance companies have "caps" on the amount they will pay for any particular medical treatment or the number of hospital days they will cover for any particular illness. Do not be afraid to check out the costs of elective procedures with the hospital or doctor. Be sure to find out how much will be covered so there are no surprises.

Many prepaid health care groups also have approved care providers. This may mean that there are restrictions on which specific doctors and hospitals you may use and still receive coverage. You should carefully check these facts out before joining one of these groups, because the doctor or hospital you have used for years may not be part of the plan. Of course, if you seek care from a nonmember, the plan will not pay unless they have specifically approved an exception for you.

Finally, if you have a child, or any family member for that matter, with a chronic illness, check very carefully before changing insurance companies. You may find that there are required waiting periods during which you will have no or only partial coverage. This may cause you a very unpleasant financial surprise.

For children who have "end-stage renal disease (ESRD)" (those receiving some form of dialysis or transplantation), the federal government has a program that assists in the payment of the medical costs. Called the Medicare ESRD program, it pays a portion of the costs of dialysis and transplantation. The formula for reimbursement is quite complicated and can change. You should consult with the nephrology social worker and/or the hospital Medicare expert to get an up-to-date explanation of the current reimbursement policies. If you have your own separate medical insurance policy, it will generally pay for much of the uncovered portion of the bills. Since the average yearly cost for dialysis and the cost for transplantation add up to tens of thousands of dollars, this federal program has saved thousands of families from financial ruin. For a child to be eligible for the Medicare program benefits, a parent must have met certain minimum eligibility requirements through the Social Security Administration. There are certain additional benefits you can receive from this Medicare program. In order to get these, you will be required to make small monthly premium payments. The social worker in your nephrology program can provide you with the details of the Medicare requirements and procedures.

In addition to the financial benefits available from insurance companies and the federal programs, there are other community financial resources generally available to kidney disease patients. These are often local or national organizations whose purpose is, in part, to provide special or emergency financial assistance to families. The specific organizations vary from region to region, although both the National Kidney Foundation and the American Kidney Fund provide resources in most areas. Above all, do not skip appointments or fail to purchase medications because of lack of insurance coverage. You must discuss such situations with your pediatric nephrologist or social worker who will work with you to resolve these problems. They can give you details on the type and extent of assistance available in particular situations.

Again, we'd like to encourage all families to find out more about the above subjects, because the specifics will differ from one state and hospital to another. There are many other important resources and bits of helpful information that can make it easier to cope with childhood kidney disease. The best way to find out about them is to ask lots of questions and be persistent in getting adequate answers.

Chapter 11
Future Horizons

A great deal of promising research in kidney disease in children involves two different, but related areas—prevention and treatment. Prevention is by far the most ideal area in which to make progress, since the prevention of kidney disease would make treatment unnecessary. However, the concept of being able to prevent all kidney disease is, at the present time, unrealistic. Therefore, the discovery of new treatments must continue to be a priority for now.

Treatment can be considered to include both 1) the treatment of disease in the child's own kidneys to minimize or stop the effects of the disease, and 2) the replacement of kidney function in those children in whom the disease has already progressed to irreversible kidney failure. Many of the techniques now under development will probably overlap the realms of both prevention and treatment.

Research in the Prevention of Kidney Disease

An effective approach to the prevention of any disease requires an understanding of its cause as well as the mechanisms by which it progresses. To the scientist, the term for cause is "etiology," and the term for the mechanism of progression is "pathogenesis." While the etiologies of some kidney diseases are quite clear, the precise cause of many hereditary kidney diseases and abnormal urinary system development is generally unknown. In cases such as polycystic kidney disease or vesicoureteral reflux, the inheritance patterns are well recognized, but the actual gene defect resulting in the abnormalities remains incompletely understood.

Current basic research in genetic structure (called gene mapping) has the potential to allow new insights into the nature of genetic processes. Through these we can expect to gain a better understanding of the inherited factors that are associated with many types of malformations. Knowledge of these genetic causes will be an important part of early diagnosis or prevention.

A different, but related, approach involves research into conditions in the environment that may produce congenital kidney disease (present at birth). These investigations focus on various physical conditions and environmental toxins that interfere with normal development. These studies are now early in the discovery process.

With the use of newer, more powerful laboratory techniques it is reasonable to expect that the relationships of substances in the environment to the development of kidney disease in the unborn child can be determined. This two-pronged approach of hereditary and environmental research holds promise for the prevention of renal disease in future generations.

For many of the so-called acquired renal diseases, the etiology and the pathogenesis are better understood. An example would be a kidney infection caused by bacteria. The growth of the bacteria in the urinary system is the etiology of the illness, and the inflammation caused by the infection is the pathogenesis of the kidney injury. The etiology and pathogenesis of kidney infections are well known, and they can be successfully treated; in many cases, recurrent infections can be prevented.

Other acquired diseases are known to have clearly defined environmental causes. A past example occurred in Britain, where the nephrotic syndrome was found to be associated with the ingestion of mercury, which was a component of a popular over-the-counter medicinal used for infants who were teething. In this case mercury toxicity was the etiology of the nephrotic syndrome, and the toxic effect of mercury on the kidney tubule was the pathogenesis of the protein loss that occurred in these infants. Removal of mercury from the medicinal was important in preventing further cases of nephrotic syndrome.

At this time one can hope that improved biochemical methods for detection of toxins in the environment will gradually determine if long-term, low-level exposure to these agents may be causing some forms of acquired kidney disease. It remains a fact, however, that many of the acquired kidney diseases, just as the inherited kidney diseases, are of unknown cause and have an unclear pathogenesis. Thus, prevention of many acquired kidney diseases also lies beyond our grasp at the present time.

Research in the Treatment of Kidney Disease

The main goal of treatment, obviously, is the elimination of the kidney problem. If that cannot be done, then treatment should be aimed at 1) preventing or minimizing further kidney damage, 2) preventing or minimizing damage to other organs because of the kidney problem, and 3) making the patient feel as good as possible. These three aims have rehabilitation of the child as their bottom-line goal. Traditionally it has been the physician's goal to help the patient live as normal a life as possible. This can be particularly challenging for the child who should be growing physically and emotionally while having to deal with kidney disease. It is further complicated by the fact that nearly all medications and treatments have some type of side effects. It is the art of medicine to optimize the child's treatment to accomplish the three goals stated above, while producing the fewest side effects possible from the treatment.

For treatment to be most effective, the kidney problem needs to be diagnosed as early as possible so that the patient can receive the treatment before irreversible kidney damage has taken place. Recently, considerable interest has developed in diagnosing certain kidney diseases in infants prior to their birth. It is reasoned that, in such cases, treatment may be instituted as soon after delivery as possible, thereby reducing the amount of kidney damage.

This approach to diagnosis before birth is called "prenatal diagnosis." Techniques such as ultrasound examination of the fetus or sampling of the amniotic fluid (amniocentesis) are being more widely used to facilitate early diagnosis. An example is the infant in whom an obstructed urinary system is diagnosed prior to birth and who may then be considered for surgical relief of the obstruction soon after delivery. This approach might prevent further kidney damage and reduce the risk of urinary infection.

It even has been suggested that surgery on the fetus while it is still in the uterus (intrauterine surgery) will become a way of producing even earlier correction of the abnormal anatomy in the future. Even for those infants who have severe kidney disease for which there is no surgical correction (such as some forms of polycystic kidney disease), early diagnosis will allow counseling of the parents prior to the delivery of the child, thereby preparing them for the problems they and their new baby will face.

Prenatal diagnosis, combined with identification of the genes responsible for the kidney malformations, may allow for reproductive counseling for couples who are at risk. It is conceivable that sometime in the future, gene manipulation will be possible so that these malformations can be eliminated altogether. At this time, however, such gene research is only just beginning.

As mentioned, the etiology of many acquired kidney diseases continues to be unknown. In spite of this, the pathogenesis of some of these illnesses or groups of illnesses is becoming more completely understood. This applies in particular to those diseases where various immune or coagulation processes are producing the ongoing kidney damage.

An example would be the kidney disease associated with the disease called "systemic lupus erythematosus." While it remains unclear what exactly triggers this illness, enough is now known of the immune processes that produce the damage so that certain medications can be used to control much of the damaging inflammation. As the immune mechanisms become even better understood in the future, it is reasonable to expect new drugs will be identified that will even more specifically target the abnormal immune reactions, stopping the disease while producing the fewest effects on other, uninvolved immune functions.

Over recent years it has become realized that the patient with kidney disease is very susceptible to the development of a "vicious circle" of kidney injury. In other words, the kidney injury may produce an abnormality (high blood pressure, for example) that, if left untreated, will go on to produce an even greater degree of kidney damage. The mechanism by which uncontrolled high blood pressure produces the kidney damage may be entirely different from the mechanism that originally caused the kidney injury. The combined effects of both injuries, however, make the kidney damage worse than either one would have alone. New therapies, including both medication and diet, are aimed at interrupting these vicious circles. In fact, there is considerable current research on the effect of various dietary components, such as protein and phosphorus, on the ongoing damage seen in many types of kidney disease. Furthermore, new drugs are constantly being developed to improve treatment of problems such as high blood pressure and high phosphorus level. These medications are very important in breaking the vicious circles of kidney damage.

Research is also very active in advancing our understanding of how kidney disease causes damage to other parts of the body. The effect of kidney disease on the growth of the body as well as the development of the brain and nervous system is of particular importance, since childhood is the time of life when most of this growth occurs. It can be expected that the administration of certain growth-producing hormones, now produced artificially in a very pure form using the new DNA technology, will be used to maximize the child's growth and development. Understanding of the mechanisms by which the rapidly growing brain of the infant or the more gradually developing brain of the child is damaged by kidney disease should lead to medications or nutritional alterations that will minimize such damage.

Other hormones produced by DNA techniques also are becoming important. A specific example is an artificial copy of the kidney hormone erythropoietin, which is normally produced by the kidney to control the production of red blood cells. The damaged kidney cannot produce this hormone, and therefore the child develops anemia. The administration of the artificial hormone to a child with kidney failure prevents the development of anemia and eliminates the need for frequent blood transfusions.

Certain kidney diseases, such as the glomerulonephritis that sometimes follows streptococcal infections or the hemolytic-uremic syndrome, will generally resolve on their own. Such diseases are said to be "self-limited." While these illnesses do go away, affected children may be very ill from kidney failure or other problems that occur during active phases of the disease. There continues to be ongoing research into medications and treatments, including dialysis, that are designed to help these patients survive their period of severe illness so that their kidney will have time to recover. In addition, artificial kidney treatment has become available even to small infants. It can be expected that such artificial kidney treatments will continue to be perfected so that they will be more easily applied and be more effective in all patients.

Finally, the area of renal replacement therapy in the form of kidney transplantation is undergoing rapid improvement because of research. New medications and approaches are being developed that help the body accept the kidney transplant, minimizing the risk of rejection. Some of these medications suppress certain aspects of the immune system so that the rejection process cannot proceed. These are called immunosuppressive medications.

A somewhat different approach involves "fooling" the immune system of the patient into thinking the transplanted kidney is a natural part of the patient and not from another individual. This approach is called "immune modulation." Many of the immune suppression medications in current use have the disadvantage of being rather broad in their effect, inhibiting good immune functions (such as protecting against infection) as well as blocking rejection. Some of the more promising new agents (such as *monoclonal antibodies*) are much more specific in their action and very pure in their composition. While these and other drugs are improvements over the older immunosuppressive medications, it is unlikely they will be the final answer.

Also of importance is the development of new drugs to combat the infections (particularly viral infections) to which transplant patients are so susceptible. The physician who manages transplant patients has always "walked a tightrope" between giving enough immunosuppression to prevent rejection, but not too much to allow infection. The new drugs that are effective against viruses, fungi, and bacterial infections now make that tightrope a little wider.

Some of the most persistent problems that remain to be solved in all of medicine, and particularly in the field of kidney disease, involve human nature. One of the most vexing is the problem of patient compliance with treatment programs. By this is meant the willingness of patients to take their medications regularly and to follow directions concerning diet, fluid intake, and activity. A large number of kidney transplant patients, including renal transplant recipients, are noncompliant. As a result, there is an unnecessary loss of successfully transplanted kidneys every year because patients stop taking their medications. This is particularly a problem with adolescent patients. Investigations into the complexities of the immune system seem simple compared to understanding human motivation.

Another problem related to human nature has to do with the availability of kidneys for transplantation. There continues to be a major shortage of donor organs. The number of persons willing to donate their kidneys if they become the unfortunate victims of accidents or other fatal events has not increased as fast as the number of persons needing kidney transplantation. It has been predicted that if the shortage of organs continues, it may be necessary to consider unrelated or distantly related living donors for kidney transplant for certain patients. This is expected to create a new set of ethical dilemmas for society, as people with less emotional attachment to the patient are asked if they would be willing to take the risk of donating one of their kidneys.

Paying Today for Tomorrow's Care and Cures

Finally a word about current research and future care. Improved care depends on a balance of basic and applied research combined with clinical investigation. Basic research often involves basic biochemistry or the use of single cells or lower animals, and to many it may appear to have no application to the problem of the child with kidney disease. Applied research tests discoveries made in basic research to see if they hold true in animals that are closer to humans in terms of kidney biology, and to see if they can be used or altered to treat a specific disease. Finally, clinical research evaluates the safety and effectiveness in humans of new treatments and procedures that have already been shown to be safe and effective in animals.

Some people object to the use of animals in research, but there simply is no other way at this time to adequately test medical discoveries before they are tried in humans. "Animal rights" groups assert that such alternatives as computers and tissue cultures could be used to replace animals, but these systems are not nearly sophisticated enough to replicate the complicated biological interactions in a human. Medical researchers are trying to reduce or replace the use of animals whenever it is possible to do so without jeopardizing important research. It would be highly unethical, however, to abandon medical research using animals, which has been a crucial part of nearly every medical advance of the 19th and

20th centuries. This would leave millions of people who are afflicted with diseases without any hope of living normal lives.

Medical research in general may seem to progress too slowly and to be both expensive and wasteful, satisfying only the trivial interest of the highly focused research scientist. However, it is those areas of basic and applied research of years past that provided the procedures and treatments on which today's clinical care is based. It would be very naive and shortsighted to restrict research only to those questions that seem to be important for today's care of the patient. Even the brightest mind cannot predict which of today's basic research projects will open the way for a dramatic new treatment for tomorrow's patient.

In these times of limited national financial resources, where there is a constant struggle for support, there has to be a far thinking, coordinated attitude toward research that will include both public and private agencies. This policy must recognize the mutual interdependence and value of basic research, applied research, and clinical research so that improved prevention and treatment will be available for our children and grandchildren. Only through such broadly based research will the promise of improved care become a reality.

Glossary

Abdomen. The part of the body between the chest and pelvis; the belly. The abdomen is lined by the peritoneal membrane, which is used in peritoneal dialysis.

Anemia. The condition resulting from decreased amounts of red blood cells, which carry oxygen to body tissues.

Aplasia. The failure of one or both kidneys to form in a developing fetus.

Artery. A blood vessel that carries blood away from the heart.

Biopsy. The removal of a piece of living tissue (for example, a sample of kidney) for diagnosis.

Bladder. The muscular sac holding urine produced by the kidneys.

Blood pressure. The pressure level in blood vessels that occurs as the heart pumps the blood through the body.

Bone marrow. A cloudy fluid contained within the cavity in the center of many bones (particularly long bones). The bone marrow is the production center for red and white blood cells and platelets.

BUN. See UREA NITROGEN.

CAPD. Abbreviation for continuous ambulatory peritoneal dialysis (see PERITONEAL DIALYSIS).

CCPD. Abbreviation for continuous cyclic peritoneal dialysis (see PERITONEAL DIALYSIS).

Catheter. A slender tube, generally made of plastic or rubber, which allows passage of fluids into or out of the body. Examples are urinary catheters, which are generally placed in the bladder, peritoneal dialysis catheters, which are placed into the abdomen, and vascular catheters, which are placed into blood vessels.

Congenital. Referring to a condition or problem existing at birth.

Creatinine. A substance normally produced from muscle cells. The level of creatinine in the blood is commonly used to estimate kidney function.

Cyst. A space or sac filled with fluid or other material. A variety of kidney diseases are associated with the formation of cysts (cystic diseases).

Cystic dysplasia. The association of cysts within the kidney with abnormal kidney development (see CYSTS, DYSPLASIA).

Cystitis. Inflammation of the bladder, most commonly the result of infection.

Dialysis. The process of passing fluid and dissolved substances across a tissue membrane. This principle forms the basis for both hemodialysis and peritoneal dialysis, where the dissolved substances that are removed include many of the body's waste products, which are present as a result of the kidney failure.

Dysplasia. Abnormal development of kidney tissue resulting in poorly formed nephron structures. If extensive, may result in poor kidney function.

Dysuria. Pain or burning sensation during urination, which is commonly associated with urinary infections.

Edema. Abnormal accumulation of fluid in a body part or cavity.

Enuresis. Inability to control urination.

Electrolytes. The term that refers to a frequently obtained laboratory test of a group of important substances: sodium, potassium, chloride, and carbon dioxide.

Erythropoietin. A hormone, made predominantly by the kidney, that stimulates the production of red blood cells.

Exchange. A single cycle of peritoneal dialysis during which the solution is passed into the abdomen and, after a period of time, drained out. Daily peritoneal dialysis usually requires a number of exchanges.

Fistula. In the case of dialysis, the direct surgical connection of an artery and vein for hemodialysis.

Glomerulonephritis. The general term referring to kidney diseases in which there is inflammation of the glomeruli.

Glomerulosclerosis. The general term referring to kidney diseases in which there is scarring of the glomeruli.

Glomerulus (plural form is glomeruli). In the kidney, the microscopic cluster of blood vessels in which blood filtration and the initial stages of urine formation occur.

Graft. The general term that refers to the transfer of tissue in the body. In the case of hemodialysis, a graft is a blood vessel made of artificial material used to connect an artery and vein (see FISTULA). A graft is also the term used to describe an organ that is transplanted.

Hematuria. The presence of blood in the urine. This blood may not be visible to the eye and may be detectable only by chemical testing (microscopic hematuria) or easily visible (gross hematuria).

Hemodialysis. The form of dialysis in which blood is passed from the body through an artificial membrane in order to remove body wastes and excessive fluid and minerals.

Hemolytic-uremic syndrome. Sudden, severe kidney failure caused by the formation of clots in the small blood vessels of the kidney and the breakdown of red blood cells.

Hereditary disease. A disease caused by a defect or defects in the genetic material received from one's parents or passed along to one's children through sexual reproduction.

Hormone. The general term referring to a substance produced in the body that has a specific effect on the activity of an organ.

Hydration. The fluid state of the body. Severe deficiency of fluid is called dehydration; excessive fluid is called overhydration.

Hypertension. The state of abnormally elevated blood pressure.

Hypoplasia. A condition in which a kidney has normally developed nephrons, but fewer than normal. If the kidneys are very small, poor function can result.

Immune system. The system having primary responsibility for protection of the body from injury caused by infectious organisms such as bacterial and viral germs. It is made up of white blood cells and chemical substances that can destroy these germs. The problems of transplant rejection largely result from this system's ability to detect what "belongs" and what "doesn't belong" within the body.

Inflammation. The condition of body tissue as a reaction to injury. This usually includes some combination of redness, heat, swelling, and tenderness, which occur to a large degree as a result of the immune system's activities.

Lipoid nephrosis. See MINIMAL CHANGE DISEASE.

Membrane. A thin layer of natural or artificial tissue. In dialysis, these membranes allow the selective passage of fluids and dissolved substances.

Mineral. One of a number of naturally occurring materials that are maintained in the body in carefully controlled concentrations. Those minerals most commonly monitored in kidney diseases include sodium, potassium, chloride, calcium, and phosphorus.

Minimal change disease. The common cause of nephrotic syndrome in children, usually beginning before 8 years of age.

Monoclonal antibody. A laboratory-produced substance that can seek out and attach to specific types of cells. Specific types of monoclonal antibodies can be used as a drug to neutralize a type of immune cell or as a diagnostic test to indicate the presence of a specific type of cell.

Nephritis. The general term referring to inflammation and disease of the kidneys (see GLOMERULONEPHRITIS).

Nephron. The individual functioning unit of the kidney, comprised of a single glomerulus, the connecting tubule, and its blood supply.

Nephrosis. See NEPHROTIC SYNDROME.

Nephrotic syndrome. The general term used to describe the condition of excessive urinary protein losses accompanied by edema.

This may occur as a disease state itself, or in association with certain forms of nephritis.

Nil disease. See MINIMAL CHANGE DISEASE.

Nuclear medicine. A specialty of medicine in which diagnostic tests are done by injecting liquids containing very low-level radioactive dyes that make body structures appear when photographed by special X-ray machines.

Parathyroid hormone. A substance produced by the parathyroid glands that helps the body process and use calcium properly.

Pass. See EXCHANGE.

Peritoneal dialysis. The form of dialysis in which fluid is passed in and out of the abdomen, during which time wastes and excessive body fluid and minerals are removed.

Peritonitis. An infection or inflammation occurring within the abdomen. This type of infection may occur in otherwise healthy children but is more frequent in those with nephrotic syndrome or patients undergoing peritoneal dialysis.

Platelets. Blood cells that are involved in blood coagulation (clotting).

Protein. The general term describing substances that are manufactured by the body and that are essential components of virtually every organ of the body. For example, they are the major constituent of cells, form the basic structure for hormones, and are the backbone of our genetic material (DNA). Specialized proteins in the body are produced from the protein contained in many foods.

Pyelonephritis. Inflammation of the kidney, generally as a result of bacterial infection (also see CYSTITIS).

Radiology. The field of medicine that uses various forms of energy (for example X rays, other forms of radiation, and sound waves) for medical diagnosis.

Red blood cells. Circulating cells of the blood whose principal role is to carry oxygen to body tissues. These tissues require oxygen to create the energy necessary to run bodily functions.

Reflux. This is more correctly called vesicoureteral reflux or urinary reflux. It is a term used to indicate the abnormal regurgitation of urine from the bladder toward the kidneys.

Rejection. The reaction of the immune system to material (a transplanted organ) that is identified as having come from another individual.

Renal. A descriptive term for something pertaining to the kidney (for example the "renal artery" or a "renal scan").

Renin. A hormone produced by the kidney and an important component of blood pressure control. Blood pressure rises when renin stimulates the production of several other hormones that cause constriction of arteries and retention of salt and water by the kidney.

SUN. See UREA NITROGEN.

Transplantation. In nephrology, the removal of a kidney from one individual and its placement into another.

Tubule. The part of the nephron that processes fluid filtered in the glomerulus, changing its composition in response to body needs and ultimately excreting it as urine.

Tunnel infection. An infection of the insertion site of a peritoneal catheter where it passes under the skin into the abdominal cavity.

Ultrafiltration. The process whereby excess water can be passed out of the body through a membrane during dialysis.

Ultrasound. A diagnostic method in which sound waves are passed through the skin and bounced off structures within the body to create pictures of organs and their internal structures.

Urea. A substance produced in the body as a result of the metabolism of proteins. Urea is a commonly measured substance that accumulates in the blood in patients with dehydration, abnormal kidney function, and several other conditions.

Urea nitrogen. A method of estimating urea. It can be measured in the blood to evaluate certain aspects of kidney function and diet.

Uremia. The state of illness resulting from the accumulation of waste materials in the body as kidney failure progresses.

Ureter. The muscular tube that contains the urine passing from the kidneys to the bladder.

Urethra. The tube that carries urine out of the bladder during urination.

Urinary tract (urinary system). The term referring to the kidneys and the urinary collecting and voiding system (kidney, pelvis, ureters, bladder, urethra).

Vascular access. The general term referring to the type of blood vessel connection used to perform hemodialysis (also see FISTULA, GRAFT, CATHETER).

Vein. A blood vessel that returns blood toward the heart.

Vesicoureteral reflux. Back flow of the urine from the bladder into the ureter and up to the kidney; a condition that can cause infection.

Vitamin D. A hormone whose active form is manufactured in the kidney. Vitamin D plays an essential role in the absorption of calcium and phosphorus from food and the control of calcium balance in the body.

White blood cells. The group of blood cells with a variety of immune and inflammatory functions.

Resources

A number of organizations can provide various types of assistance to patients and their families. The specific types of assistance available may vary from community to community. Nonetheless, this most often includes financial help, patient and parent support and information groups, educational programs, and printed material on a variety of topics. The social workers serving the nephrology patient are generally knowledgeable about the resources in your area. Your child need not have "end-stage renal disease" before you seek out the dialysis social worker for this type of advice.

Since many foundations and medical institutions produce their own publications and brochures for their patients, it is impossible to accurately compile lists of such materials that might be available. Two services may help this situation. First is the National Kidney and Urologic Diseases Information Clearinghouse (NKUDIC). The NKUDIC was established by the National Institute of Diabetes and Digestive and Kidney Diseases of the National Institutes of Health. Its goal is to provide an information resource about kidney and urologic diseases to patients, health workers, and the public. The clearinghouse can respond to specific inquiries as well as providing lists of published materials. You can contact them at the following address and telephone number:

Box NKUDIC
Bethesda, MD 20892
(301) 468-6345

Two journals may also provide useful information. The journal *Urologic Nursing* publishes a list of booklets and fact sheets about a variety of urologic disorders. Most of these materials have been produced at medical institutions that are willing to make them available to the general public. *Urologic Nursing* is published by The American Urological Association Allied, Inc. (editorial offices at 9432 Southwest 12th Drive, Portland, OR 97219). The journal of the Association for the Care of Children's Health, *Children's Health Care,* publishes material pertaining to health care issues in pediatrics. While not a specific journal for patients with kidney disorders, it contains articles that might have general usefulness for children with chronic illnesses.

The National Kidney Foundation and the American Kidney Fund are two organizations that provide a variety of direct patient services as well as serving as information resources for patients. The American Kidney Fund can provide small grants to families with financial crises. It also has a number of pamphlets available for patients. You can write to the AKF at:

7315 Wisconsin Ave.
Suite 203 E
Bethesda, MD 20814-3266
(800) 638-8299

The National Kidney Foundation provides services that include educational and support programs as well as some financial aid. This varies considerably among local Kidney Foundation affiliates depending upon local resources and needs. It is best to contact your closest Kidney Foundation Affiliate and inquire about programs in your area. You can also contact the National Office directly at:

30 East 33rd St.
New York, NY 10016
(800) 622-9010

Last, but certainly not least, are the patient organizations. The American Association of Kidney Patients has a growing number of chapters nationally. The AAKP publishes pamphlets, brochures, and a journal, conducts seminars and has been active in a number of related kidney disease organizations. It also is an active self-advocacy organization, lobbying to protect the interests of kidney patients. For information and membership inquiries, write or call:

American Association of Kidney Patients
1 Davis Boulevard
Suite LL-1
Tampa, FL 33606
(813) 251-0725

In addition, the Polycystic Research Foundation is a patient organization with a more specific focus. For more information about their activities and materials, you can contact this group at:

922 Walnut St.
Kansas City, MO 64106
(816) 421-1869

Several selected publications of particular interest to children and/or their families include:

1. *Bouncy Bunny's Birthday: A Family Story about Bravery.* By C. Brown, M.S.W., and D. Patterson, R.N. A book intended to assist parents in helping children express their feelings about chronic illness.
   Creative Expressions
   PO Box 456
   Colchester, VT 05446

2. *Countdown for Takeoff.* By National Kidney Foundation, Inc. A kit of activity books and logs which was designed to introduce pediatric patients to life on dialysis as they begin this treatment.

    National Kidney Foundation, Inc.
    (See address above.)

3. *Diet for Patients with Renal Failure.* By National Kidney Foundation of Texas, Inc. (also available in Spanish). An overview of nutritional considerations for patients on peritoneal dialysis.

    National Kidney Foundation of Texas, Inc.
    3500 Midway Road, Suite 101
    Dallas, TX 75234

4. *Even in Heaven They Don't Sing All the Time.* Edited by Connie Jones, A.C.S.W. An inspiring book of articles edited by a renal social worker and written by kidney patients and their families about day-to-day coping with kidney failure and its treatment.

    National Kidney Foundation of Georgia, Inc.
    1899 Screwart Ave.
    Atlanta, GA 30309
    (404) 755-3443

5. *Family Focus.* By National Kidney Foundation, Inc. A quarterly newsletter published for dialysis and transplant patients and their families. Many of the articles offer interesting and helpful points of view, many of which are pertinent to children and their families.

    National Kidney Foundation, Inc.
    (See address above.)

6. *Someone Special. How Mike Learns to Live with Kidney Disease.* Edited by Glenn H. Bock, M.D., and Marshall G. Hoff. A children's book written by children's writers and illustrators about a child and his parents who experience, for the first time, doctors and nurses in a hospital during a kidney disease evaluation.

    University of Minnesota
    Department of Pediatrics, Box 491
    Division of Pediatric Nephrology
    Minneapolis, MN 55455

Index

Glenn H. Bock, M.D., is vice chairman of the Department of Pediatric Nephrology, Children's National Medical Center, and associate professor of pediatrics, the George Washington University School of Medicine, both in Washington, D.C. He has recently completed a research sabbatical at the National Institute of Health and has authored more than fifty scientific articles, abstracts, and textbook chapters. He has had a long-standing interest in both professional and patient education, and has served on regional and national research, education, and patient service committees for the National Kidney Foundation.

Edward J. Ruley, M.D., is chairman of the Department of Pediatric Nephrology at Children's National Medical Center, and professor of pediatrics at the George Washington University School of Medicine.

Michael P. Moore has been a science writer for ten years and is now director of communications for the Office of Research and Technology Transfer Administration at the University of Minnesota. He has also coauthored books about diabetes and epilepsy.